The
evenflo®
Guide to
Breastfeeding

Library of Congress Cataloging in Publication Data

Main entry under title:

The Evenflo guide to breastfeeding.

1. Breast feeding. I. Evenflo Juvenile Products Co.
II. Title: Guide to breastfeeding.
RJ216.E83 1984   649'.3   84-6094
ISBN 0-937558-05-2

Text prepared and book designed by
Robert Scharff and Associates, Ltd.

10   9   8   7   6   5   4   3   2   1

Printed in the United States of America

CONTENTS

Chapter 1   Making the Decision 1

Chapter 2   Preparing for Breastfeeding 20

Chapter 3   Beginning to Nurse 32

Chapter 4   The Number One Priority—
             Take Care of Yourself 54

Chapter 5   Substances That May Affect You
             and Your Baby 73

Chapter 6   Breastfeeding While Working 82

Chapter 7   When Problems Arise 99

Chapter 8   Changing Nutritional Needs 111

We would like to thank the following companies and institutions for supplying some of the photographs that appear in this book: Mead Johnson & Company; Pottsville Hospital and Warne Clinic, Pottsville, PA; and the High Risk Nursery Staff of Welborn Baptist Hospital, Evansville, IN. In addition, we would like to express our appreciation to certain groups and companies for their assistance and/or use of their products: Discovery Workshop Daycare Center, Schuylkill Haven, PA, and the Questor Juvenile Furniture Company.

ADVISORY BOARD

1
Making the Decision

Feeding your baby is one of the most rewarding and important responsibilities you assume when you become a parent. During the first few months of life, food means everything to your baby. It soothes tummy aches, provides energy to kick and wriggle, and is accompanied by your warm embrace. However, it's not only food, but the *right type* of food that is essential.

Consider that when you stroll into the kitchen for a midnight snack, you are in total control of what and when you eat. But what about the baby you are expecting? Babies cannot fend for themselves. Why they couldn't even reach the refrigerator door handle if they wanted to! No, it's going to be your responsibility as parents to take complete charge of your baby's nutrition—to be both cook and waiter. But what should you feed your baby?

For the first six months, either breast milk or formula should be the sole item on your baby's menu. But which is best? As a friend of the family, Evenflo wants to help you make this very important decision. That's why we've written this book, *The Evenflo Guide to Breastfeeding*. By the time you're through reading, you'll have a good idea why "breast may be best" for your baby. It's natural, it's nutritious, and it's a nice way to start off your baby's life.

Changing Trends

Since no bottles have been found in archeological digs, we can assume that breastfeeding has been insuring the survival of the human race for a very long time. Now this doesn't mean that all mothers nursed their own babies. In ancient times, wealthy women would hire professional "nursers" to take over feeding duties. But even though these mothers did not do their nursing themselves, they did know the value of breast milk.

In fact, breast milk was considered so vital throughout the centuries that it became the subject of many myths, stories, and works of art. For example, according to mythology, breast milk gave the mighty Hercules his immortality. Hercules' father, Zeus, King of the Gods, placed his infant at the breast of the sleeping goddess Juno. After Hercules had stopped nursing, Juno's milk continued to flow. Some drops fell to earth and were transformed into clusters of milky white lilies. Still more breast milk drifted throughout the sky, forming what we now call the Milky Way. Painters have also relished in depicting nursing mothers, including illustrations of the tale we have just related. The mothers shown are black as well as white, their nationalities and backgrounds varied, but all serve as a testament to the importance of this age-old practice.

The Birth of the Bottle. If breastfeeding has been around so long, then how does one account for the popularity of the bottle? Its success had a great deal to do with the changing role of women in society. In the early 1900s when it was introduced, bottlefeeding revolutionized baby care. This was the time when women were becoming liberated from the home—they were bobbing their hair, shortening their skirts, and stepping out in the world of men. The bottle became part of this revolution; it represented freedom from the traditional ties of motherhood.

Of course, not all women became trendsetters. For those who were poor, uneducated, and newly arrived in America, there was no escape from the home. As was traditional, the husband went out and worked while his hard-pressed wife stayed home and cared for her babies—in addition to scrubbing clothes on a washboard, hauling coal for the stove, and perhaps feeding 10 to 15 boarders. Yet these women, too, adopted bottlefeeding. It freed them to take care of other tasks, while allowing them to somewhat mimic mothers of the upper class. Soon, virtually every mother was bottlefeeding her baby—it was the thing to do. Breastfeeding implied poverty and poor education. Even physicians literally forgot that nursing had ever existed.

Back to the Breast. Although formulas remain popular to this day, the majority of pediatricians are again recommending breastfeeding as the best way to nourish a baby. Besides the fact that breast milk is the ideal infant food, the act of nursing benefits you, the mother, as well. As a result of such endorsements, infant feeding trends are again changing. In 1955 only 30% of mothers breastfed their babies and most were weaned before they were two months old. That figure rose to 71% in 1983 and is still on the increase.

Despite this growing phenomenon, however, you and many other women may never have seen a nursing mother. And while there now are numerous groups promoting breastfeeding, you may not have been exposed to much of their material or may be hesitant to contact them for fear they'll consider your questions to be silly. Your husband, too, may be concerned about whether breastfeeding is best for his child and may be reluctant to give his wholehearted support to the idea. Because of this, your mind may understandably be filled with doubts about breastfeeding: Will it make me fat? Can I still work? To what extent will it tie me down?

Questions similar to these may have peaked your interest in breastfeeding, or a friend may have introduced you to the idea. Now, in addition, you know a bit about the historical aspects of breastfeeding. "But when," you may be wondering, "am I going to find out any concrete facts?" In the following sections and throughout the remainder of this book, you'll learn all you need

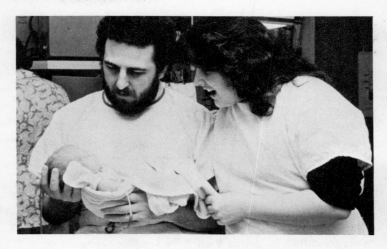

to know to comfortably breastfeed your baby—from how it works to how to work while nursing. So read on and remain in suspense no longer.

Why Breast Milk?

Breast milk has no substitutes or stand-ins. It's species specific; that is, the milk of every species is different and unique. Human milk is made for human babies, just as cow's milk is the perfect food for calves. It has precisely the right combination of nutrients, plus numerous other advantages as well. No matter how near formulas come to simulating breast milk, they're just not the same. And untreated cow's milk, once another popular alternative to breast milk, is now considered nutritionally unsuitable for baby's first year. Does this mean you must breastfeed for an entire year? Not really; your baby can eventually be weaned to a formula with no ill effects. But the longer you continue to nurse, the more benefits your baby will receive.

Better Nutrition

Breast milk is the most nutritionally complete food for your baby. While human milk does vary in exact composition from mother to mother—even in one mother from night to day—it still fulfills all your baby's needs. (See Chapter 2.) Premature babies frequently do well on breast milk, but poorly on formula. For more information on caring for a premature baby, refer to *The Evenflo Guide to Your Baby's Health from birth to one year.*

Readily Digestible

Because breast milk is relatively dilute and contains a special type of protein, it is readily and easily digested. Breast milk promotes the growth of desirable bacteria in your baby's digestive system, leading to fewer instances of diarrhea and constipation. In general, breastfed babies usually have fewer digestive disorders, upset stomachs, and cases of colic, making life much more peaceful for you, too.

Resistance to Disease

Medical records have shown that babies breastfed for four and one-half months or longer are two to three times less susceptible to many childhood diseases, including respiratory infections. Breast milk, particularly the first milk, or *colostrum*, gives your baby temporary immunities to diseases an infant might be exposed to shortly after birth. Colostrum contains *antibodies*, or immunity carriers, as well as *macrophages* and many other agents that protect the digestive tract from bacteria and allergies.

Fewer Allergies

Allergic reaction to breast milk is an extreme rarity. Cow's milk-based and soy-based formulas are often at the root of such disorders, especially if you or your husband has a history of allergy problems. Breastfed babies have less chance of developing eczema and other common skin rashes, asthma, and allergic runny nose, and experience fewer instances of vomiting and fitfulness.

Purity

The possibility of spoilage or contamination of breast milk is extremely remote, although your baby may be affected by your use of alcohol, cigarettes, or drugs. (See Chapter 5.)

Natural Pacification

Your breasts not only give baby milk, but serve to soothe and comfort, too! Pacifiers work well on some occasions, but they aren't warm and soft like your breasts are when your baby is snuggled close in your arms. For a baby, anything else is second best.

Benefits for You

Ready, set, contract! Breastfeeding after delivery helps your uterus regain its pre-pregnancy size and tone. These contractions are caused by the same hormones that control milk flow, which is why you may feel them commence when your baby starts to nurse. In addition, breastfeeding speeds weight loss by using up the fat reserves accumulated during pregnancy, provided that your energy intake is appropriate.

Convenience. Breast milk is always ready and at the correct temperature, as opposed to sterile formulas that have been poured directly into a bottle but still require some preparation. With breast milk, there's no paraphernalia necessary, no need to worry about running to the store in bad weather, and no waste. This convenience also holds true when you have to travel with baby. Since less time is spent in preparation, you can devote more attention to your newborn or to other family members.

Your husband will likewise appreciate the simplicity of breastfeeding. Plus, there's no cleanup or clutter. Naturally, the

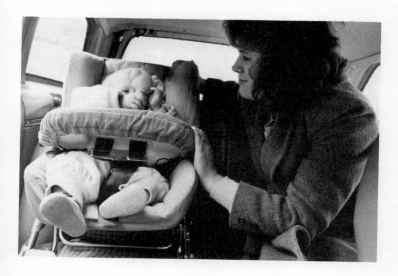

increased time you'll be able to spend together as a family will garner his "yea" vote as well.

No Overfeeding. A breastfed baby is in complete control of food intake because the sucking regulates the amount. When satisfied, your baby simply stops sucking. This self-control may avoid a tendency toward becoming overweight or obese later.

"But how can I tell if my baby is getting enough milk?" If your baby isn't, it's a rarity. Babies understand their own wants and needs better than we think. The only time they may not get enough is if a problem arises in early lactation.

Bonding. The skin-to-skin contact and time spent with your newborn while nursing results in a special relationship. How can't it, with your baby gazing contentedly up into your eyes as he or she nurses? Nursing mothers also seem to talk more to their babies, becoming more attuned to their wants and feelings.

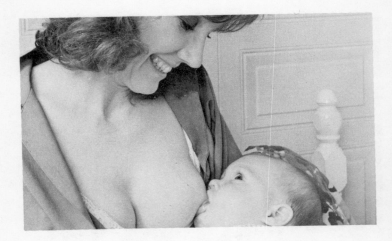

These deep emotional ties that form are termed *bonding*. When thinking about bonding, don't forget to include baby's father. While he can't actually nurse the baby, he can become part of the whole emotional experience just by being there.

Relaxation. As a new mother, your body needs time to recover from the strains of pregnancy and birth. Nursing forces you to take time out from your hectic routine to spend quiet, uninterrupted moments with your baby. The calming effects of nursing plus the knowledge that you are needed by your baby may help relieve *postpartum*, or after-birth, blues.

Deterrents to Breastfeeding

We're the first to admit that breastfeeding isn't for everyone. If we all had the same personalities, the world would be a pretty boring place. Some women want to breastfeed and others simply don't; there's nothing wrong with that. If you're straddling the fence, however, a little more sound information on breastfeeding may help you make up your mind.

Physical Factors

There are certain situations when your doctor may discourage you from breastfeeding. If this is the case, there is no need to feel guilty; that is, it's merely a fact that must be accepted. If a woman has been seriously ill during pregnancy, nursing may impose too great a strain. Mothers with highly infectious or debilitating diseases or those on certain medications that could be harmful if passed on to the baby may also be counseled to bottlefeed.

Your baby's physical condition is another factor that may determine whether or not you can nurse. A cleft palate is one good example of a problem that could hamper baby's sucking ability (though babies with cleft palate can be trained to suck at the breast if handled patiently). Premature babies may have special problems requiring the use of formulas; however, most neonatal intensive care units are now encouraging the feeding of expressed breast milk, enabling the mother to begin breastfeeding once the baby has recovered.

Limits on Freedom

A newborn may need to feed 8 to 10 times a day. And that can seem pretty scary if you are looking forward to resuming your pre-pregnancy life-style. If you are very set against being "tied down," bottlefeeding, where your husband or other family members can help with the feedings, may be the best option for you. A woman who nurses grudgingly may do more harm than good. Tensions and negative feelings pass readily to your baby, making baby uncomfortable as well.

However, for the first few months, both breastfeeding and bottlefeeding are somewhat limiting. Your body is still recovering from pregnancy, the house is more than likely in disarray, and your baby requires a fair amount of attention outside of feeding. Plus, while the initial number of breastfeedings is high, it will drop once your baby gets on a schedule. Trying to breastfeed, even for a short period after coming home from the hospital, would be beneficial for you both, giving your baby initial immunities and making you take needed time for rest. Just start out and take one day at a time.

Social Pressures

Although the practice of breastfeeding is growing rapidly, public acceptance of it varies. Many people, usually adults, are still extremely uncomfortable at the sight of a nursing mother. Part of this may be due to the sexual connotation today's society attaches to the breast. What happens if you are caught in a public place and it's feeding time?

With today's new styles of nursing bras and maternity fashions, nursing in public isn't as traumatic as it used to be; a nursing mother no longer has to expose her breast. A properly wrapped scarf or blanket can conceal the fact that baby is nursing. No one, not even your husband, may realize it! (Also try using a little discretion in where you nurse.) If you feel wary and uncertain, practice in front of a mirror until you develop a technique. By that time, though, you may find that much of your initial embarrassment has subsided.

Your Husband Can Help. While your husband, too, may be a little uncertain about the thought of his wife "baring her breasts" in public, his desire to provide the best possible nutrition for his child should enable him to support your efforts. He can help a great deal by acting as a buffer between you and uninformed people who may question or criticize your decision to breastfeed. A simple, "I'm proud to watch my wife breastfeed our child" goes a long way in putting a halt to unsolicited opinions, not to mention that it makes you feel pretty special, too!

Return to Work

"I plan to return to work soon after my baby is born!" That's the goal many career-minded mothers set for themselves.

Others, though they may not want to return to their jobs so quickly, must do so for financial reasons. Breastfed babies nurse approximately every one and one-half to three hours for the initial one to two months, making breastfeeding seem impossible to integrate with an eight-hour workday. But this really isn't the case. Breastfeeding and working can go hand-in-hand. In-house day-care, taking the baby with you, and expressing (manually removing) breast milk are all viable possibilities. (See Chapter 6.) Older babies can be partially weaned to formula for the missed feedings.

Negative Feelings of Husbands and Family Members
The knowledge that they won't have to get up in the middle of a chilly night to feed the baby is relished by some fathers. But to others who desire an active role in their baby's life, it can be extremely disturbing. They view breastfeeding as a way to exclude or exile them from their child. If this description fits your husband, you must take pains to reassure him that breastfeeding will not affect his paternal role. Suggest other ways he can help: giving bottles of expressed breast milk, bathing, accompanying you during night feedings, changing diapers, or just cuddling. Fathering is a time to let down that outward wall of reserve. Another thing you can do is make sure that he is well-informed about the advantages of breastfeeding. Unless you've already begun childbirth classes, he's probably very much confused and in the dark about the entire subject.

Changes in Your Relationship as Husband and Wife. Besides getting used to the idea of becoming a father, your husband has the additional responsibility of caring for you while you recuperate. It's a time when he may have to give more to you emotionally than he gets in return. As a result, he may become jealous. He may find it difficult to share you with the baby. Breastfeeding may intensify this reaction due to the close bonding between the nursing couple, bonding that may become so intense that you begin to view your baby as the center of your life.

All in all for your husband, your entire marital relationship may become one big blur.

Breastfeeding should not take away from your sex life or the affection you and your husband share. Rather, it should help mold you into a family. You are both making sacrifices for your baby—you by nursing and he by sharing this person who was once solely his.

Once your husband understands that he is not in competition with the baby, his feelings may quickly soften. This may also occur once he realizes how vital his support is to your success at breastfeeding and general well-being, and that negative comments from him can temporarily affect your ability to nurse. Parenting—and breastfeeding—must be a joint effort. Rather than ignoring him, let him know that you need him more than ever. You may not always verbalize your feelings, but he will read them in your eyes as you give your all to nurse his child. To help him adjust, plan time for just the two of you to be alone, even if it's only a walk around the block. Show him that the intimacy you both shared in the past hasn't disappeared, rather it's merely taken on a different "family" form.

Handling Older Children. Husbands aren't the only ones to suffer from jealousy. Your older children, too, may become alarmed at the sight of this new squawking bundle who's stealing away their mother's time and affection. They may view the intrusion more strongly if they were also breastfed.

Prepare your children for what lies ahead before the baby is born. Explain to them, as much as they can understand, about babies, but don't misinform them—no storks and no cabbage patches. Older children can attend sibling classes, where they come to the hospital and participate in group discussions on what to expect. Having your other children visit you and the new baby in the hospital can also help.

But even if they've been prepared, don't be surprised if once the baby is home your two- to five-year-old starts thumb sucking,

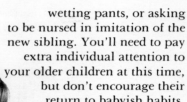

wetting pants, or asking to be nursed in imitation of the new sibling. You'll need to pay extra individual attention to your older children at this time, but don't encourage their return to babyish habits. Give them the opportunity to help with simple baby care tasks; this makes them feel important. But while allowing them to help, never leave a child between one and one-half and three years old alone with a baby. They are too young to comprehend a baby's fragility and unintentionally may harm the infant.

As far as breastfeeding is concerned, don't shoo your other children away at nursing time. They should view breastfeeding as something natural. Involve them by reading aloud to them while you breastfeed the baby. You may look up one day to find them nursing their "babies," too!

Putting Worries to Rest

All right, you've learned to handle how others may react to your decision to breastfeed. Then why are you still uncertain? Oh, you've heard some of the breastfeeding myths that are circulating—that you "need big breasts" or that you "must eat for two"—and they have you concerned. Well, then let's relegate them to their proper places as well.

Can I Nurse? At some time most mothers have doubts about their nursing ability, even if they've nursed babies before.

If you're healthy, there's no reason you can't breastfeed your baby. Age is also no deterrent. (See *The Evenflo Guide to Parenting After Thirty*.) Failures and physical inability are rare. Even a cesarean will have no effect; your milk will come in just as quickly. With knowledge and support, nursing can be a successful and enjoyable family affair.

Does My Small Breast Size Matter? The size and shape of your breasts, as well as your overall physical size, have no bearing on the quality or quantity of milk produced. Breast size is determined by fatty tissues that don't come into play in milk production. What matters is the extent of the network of milk carrying vessels and ducts, which any woman can develop. Slightly built women with small breasts often turn out to be the most successful breastfeeders.

Inverted nipples may present a problem, but they can be drawn out with special exercises or through the use of nipple shields. (See Chapter 2.)

Will Nursing Affect My Figure? Naturally, you are not thrilled about the possibility of postpartum or breastfeeding sag. Your breasts will become enlarged and heavier during lactation (milk production). But any permanent change is actually the result of heredity, maturity, and the weight gained during pregnancy. Generally, the more weight you gain, the more pendulous your breasts may become. By wearing a good, supportive nursing bra and watching your weight, however, you should experience little or no sagging.

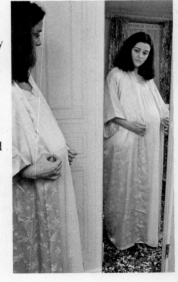

As for the rest of your figure, breastfeeding does not mean that you have to eat for two. You only need between 500 and 1,000 extra calories each day and these will be burned up in milk production. The energy is used to synthesize the milk as well as for the milk itself. Increased liquid intake is also a must, but this could be in the form of water, which will not add to your calorie count. In fact, nursing may enable you to return to your normal weight much more rapidly than would otherwise be the case.

How Can I Tell if My Baby Is Getting Enough Milk? If your baby has good color, sleeps well, and has approximately six or more wet diapers daily and pale urine, you can be fairly sure that baby is getting enough milk. Frequency of bowel movements may vary from several a day to one in four or five days.

Don't worry if your breastfed baby doesn't gain weight at first. Many babies initially lose 10% of their birth weight before it stabilizes and they begin to gain. This is in no way an effect of insufficient milk intake. Advocates of bottlefeeding may point to a chubby bottlefed baby, remarking that with formula you can always tell how much your baby is drinking. It's true that you can tell the amount baby is taking in, but a bottle doesn't tell you how much your infant "needs." The chubbiness may be the result of unintentional overfeeding and in no way indicates a healthy baby.

It's also not unusual for a breastfed baby to seem very hungry and need more frequent feedings. Because breast milk is so easily digested, baby's stomach empties more frequently and so your infant needs to feed more often.

Will I Have Enough Milk? Mother Nature takes care of this problem. The more your baby nurses, the more your milk production will increase. In other words, supply increases with demand. You can further stimulate lactation by making sure both breasts are fully emptied at each feeding. Cases where it does seem that a mother lacks milk are due to unwarranted anxiety or lack of proper encouragement, help, fluid intake, or rest.

After two to three weeks, you may notice that your baby seems dissatisfied at the breast. This is because baby's appetite is increasing not, as is often mistakenly assumed, because your supply is decreasing. Another similar growth spurt may occur around 14 weeks. More frequent feedings will increase your supply and soon have baby happy again.

Will My Milk Be Rich Enough? The appearance of breast milk has no bearing on the quality. Breast milk is normally thin (for the first part of any feeding) and skimmed looking, often with a bluish tinge. This wateriness, however, may have led your mother or grandmother to believe that the family produces poor milk.

Can My Baby Miss a Feeding? An occasional supplemental bottle won't really hurt. Do try not to interrupt the nursing pattern until lactation is firmly established. This may take about three to four weeks.

Is Rest Important? If you are tense, nervous, or overtired, improper rest will affect your milk production. Your feelings of anxiety can also be passed on, making your baby irritable as well.

Natural Infertility—Fact or Myth?

This discussion brings us to another breastfeeding legend, that of natural infertility. During pregnancy, your body hormones change, signaling the lining of your womb to build up rather than be discharged each month. This cessation of menstruation is called *pregnancy amenorrhea*. According to theory, a woman who is breastfeeding her baby can retain this infertility for a lengthy period after birth as well.

How does it work? Advocates of natural infertility, or *lactation amenorrhea*, claim that the infant must be receiving 100% of his nourishment from the breast. This means no supplemental feedings, not even water. The sucking stimulus supposedly keeps up the hormone production, preventing ovulation (release of an egg from the ovary) and thus pregnancy.

The second question—does it work? Natural infertility does occur in some women, but it is *no insurance against pregnancy* and is not totally supported by medical findings. You can't be sure when you are ovulating, and pregnancy can occur without the visible sign of menstruation. So before using this natural method of child spacing, you and your husband should consult a doctor. The physician may recommend the use of some barrier-type contraceptive as an extra precaution.

The Decision

Now that you've learned what breastfeeding is all about, you probably can't wait to get started. But do discuss it with your husband one more time to get his input. After all, it's his baby, too! You say he's convinced about breastfeeding as well? Great—you're off to a good start. By the way, if your baby had a say in the matter, there would be another "yea" vote for breastfeeding, too!

Finalizing Plans

Now that you've made your commitment to breastfeed your baby, it's important for you to inform your doctor and the hospital personnel of your decision. Becoming familiar with their ideas on breastfeeding before birth can prevent unpleasant confrontations later. You should also schedule a prenatal visit or interview with your baby's doctor to assess attitudes and procedures.

The Hospital. How successful your initial breastfeeding experiences are depends somewhat on your hospital's rules and procedures. Before you actually go in to have your baby, discuss with your doctor every aspect of the facility's maternity routine. Your labor coach—your husband or a friend—should also be present since this person will be assisting with the birth. Make it a particular point to find out how any of the medications used may affect your ability to breastfeed right after birth, or ask if they conduct natural childbirth. If some practices come in direct opposition to your wishes, make your preference known. Hospitals, in general, are becoming more relaxed in their maternity programs and may respect your request with little or no fuss if it does not jeopardize your health or your baby's.

Remind your doctor to tell those attending you that you will be breastfeeding and that you should be given no drugs to dry up milk or to contract your uterus. Also inform the nurses that your baby should receive no supplementary bottles and that baby should be brought to you for each feeding. If this is inconvenient, ask if you can go to the nursery.

The hospital can be supportive of nursing procedures by providing a relaxed atmosphere and allowing you and your baby to be together as much as possible during the hospital stay. This gives the nursing couple ample opportunity to get to know each other and be able to nurse on a schedule. Hospitals with rooming-in and nursery facilities give you an option if you need to be by yourself for a while. Many hospitals also provide breast-

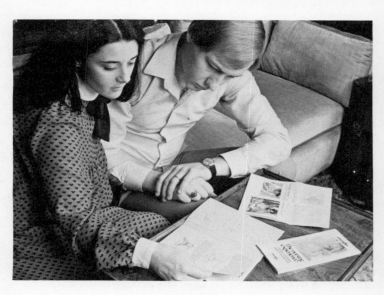

feeding rooms right in the nursery so that sick and premature infants can be comfortably breastfed as well.

Becoming Informed

You should also try to find out as much about breastfeeding as you can prior to your baby's birth. Medical personnel, relatives, and friends who have successfully breastfed their babies are all good sources of advice. So is your local La Leche League (LLL). Begun in 1956 by several mothers, the LLL, which works in support of the practice of breastfeeding, has expanded across the United States and into 43 other countries. For both you and your husband's benefit, there are also childbirth classes and parent support groups, which serve as excellent forums for breastfeeding queries.

Finally, as a friend of the family, we at Evenflo hope that we can do our part to help you throughout your breastfeeding period—to get you off to a good start and help you have a healthy, happy baby. So let's begin and explore the many joys of breastfeeding together.

2
Preparing for Breastfeeding

Throughout the months of your pregnancy, your breasts experience a series of changes that prepares them for *lactation*, or milk production. Here's what happens.

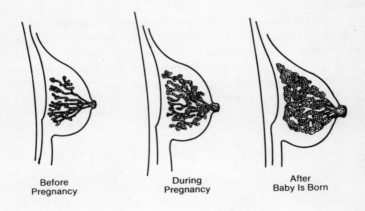

Before Pregnancy

During Pregnancy

After Baby Is Born

Your Breasts

First off, in order to feel comfortable with breastfeeding, it is essential that you become familiar with your breasts and how they function. Your breasts have three main parts: the breast, the areola, and the nipple.

The main part of your breast is composed of three types of tissue. Glandular tissue produces milk and provides the means to transport it to your hungry baby. In actuality, your breasts are nothing more than enlarged glands. Supporting connective tissue prevents sagging and gives support, while the amount of protective fatty tissue you have determines your breast size. Remember that size has nothing whatsoever to do with your ability to produce milk.

Your *areolae* are the darker, pigmented areas, or rings, surrounding your nipples. The areola contains lubricating glands and also serves as a grasping point when your baby nurses. Breast milk is exuded through approximately 15 to 20 openings in your *nipples*, the center, protruding parts of your breasts. Your nipples are well-supplied with blood vessels and nerve endings which cause them to become erect with stimulation—a response that simplifies baby's nursing.

Early Changes

During the first few weeks of pregnancy, your nipples and particularly your areolae will begin to darken. Some brunettes may experience darkening of the entire breast. The coloring will fade after birth, but never completely returns to its pre-pregnancy lightness. The darkening of the areola may act to attract baby's attention during nursing since this is the area that must be taken into baby's mouth.

A second change comes in the Montgomery's glands. These are the little pimple-like bumps found on the areola. With the onset of pregnancy, these glands enlarge and begin producing a substance that helps keep your nipples clean and lubricated.

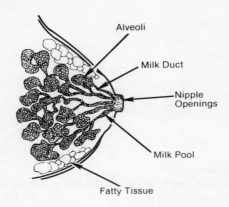

Alveoli

Milk Duct

Nipple Openings

Milk Pool

Fatty Tissue

Soaps can interfere with this natural moisturizing process and that is why it is important that you limit cleansing to rinsing your breasts.

Milk Apparatus. Directly behind your areola are the milk sinuses, or *pools,* that collect the breast milk. Branching out from these pools, like limbs on a tree, are numerous, tiny ducts that serve as passageways for the milk.

At about six weeks into your pregnancy, the ends of the ducts enlarge into sacs called *alveoli* that are lined with the cells that will produce your milk. You may also hear the alveoli referred to as the mammary, or breast, glands. You've always had the ability to produce milk. Even babies sometimes drip milk from their nipples as a result of hormones released at birth; however, it takes some stimulus to put the system into action. As the alveoli enlarge, they begin to replace some of the normal fatty tissue, resulting in the overall increase in your breast size.

Second Half of Pregnancy

When the placenta has developed, it signals your body to start production of a hormone called *prolactin*—a prolactation hormone. Prolactin stimulates the alveoli to secrete milk.

By your fourth or fifth month and at least by your sixth, the cells in the center of the alveoli undergo fatty degeneration to form the colostrum, or early milk. This clear, slightly yellowish liquid begins draining from the glands through the network of ducts and collects in the milk pools. You may experience some leaking of colostrum during the last few weeks prior to birth or even in mid-pregnancy. Don't be alarmed if it comes from the glands around the areolae as well as from the nipples. This is nothing unusual. Should your baby come prematurely, even at the beginning of the last trimester, you will be physically capable of breastfeeding.

Production Continues. As the time of your baby's birth draws near, your breasts will become fuller and firmer, partially due to the increased amount of blood in the vessels of the alveoli. You may even experience some initial discomfort or engorgement. (See Chapter 7.) Early nursing in the hospital will usually bring quick relief, but your doctor may advise you to express a few drops of colostrum for your continued comfort until the baby arrives.

Nursing Time Is Here

We've discussed your role in lactation, but what about your baby's? As you prepare to nurse, your baby's sucking stimulates the nerve endings in your nipples. In turn, these nerves send a message to your brain (to the pituitary gland) to secrete two hormones—prolactin and oxytocin. As mentioned, prolactin is responsible for the actual milk production. *Oxytocin* is the hormone responsible for orgasm, labor contractions, and the uterine cramps you experience when nursing. For some women, it also brings a relaxed, soothed feeling conducive to mothering. At this stage after birth, oxytocin causes the rubber-band-like muscles around the alveoli to contract and squeeze milk into the ducts and to the pools where it is available for your baby. This contracting is better known as the *let-down reflex.*

The Let-Down Reflex

You'll find that the contractions are anything but a let-down, so whence the name? Let-down was originally a term applied to the ability of cows to let down their milk. In England, the same reaction is called the "draught" (pronounced *draft*) and has also been labeled the "milk ejection reflex."

How can you tell if you are letting down? The most common signal is a tingling sensation in your breasts. This has been likened to a pleasant case of pins and needles. The uterine cramps, or contractions, we've mentioned are another sign. Also look for milk dripping from your nipple or a spurt of milk from the side you are not nursing. Yes, the pressure in the milk pools can spray your milk up to a foot away when stimulation occurs! Usually, however, women just have a fine spray and some may not experience this phenomenon at all.

It Takes Time. *What's taking my let-down so long?* you may be thinking. But don't worry. If you are a new mother, it may take anywhere from a few seconds to several minutes for your milk to reach the pools. In the meantime, your baby may be acting cranky or making your nipples tender through unsuccessful sucking. You can speed let-down by hand expressing a few drops (see Chapter 6), taking a warm shower, or applying warm, moist compresses. In time, it will become an almost immediate, conditioned response; that is, your milk may come in merely at the sound of your baby's cry. It can even occur due to the excitement of sexual intercourse. Women who have previously breast-fed have a quicker let-down because their milk duct network is already quite developed. If let-down continues to be a problem, your doctor may prescribe an oxytocin spray. These sprays, administered nasally, speed the reaction.

When Your Baby Nurses

Babies and breastfeeding were made for each other. Even a baby's initial physical formation is conducive to taking the breast. Babies have fatty pads in their cheeks that prevent the cheeks from caving in as the baby sucks. Those cute, chubby cheeks really do have a function! A baby's nose is short and flat, which helps an infant breathe while nursing. (Some babies need additional help in this department.) And to get at the milk, baby's ridged gums allow for a better hold on the areola.

How Your Baby Gets Milk. Your baby doesn't actually suck your milk as you might suppose. The only function of the suction is to keep the nipple in place, which babies do by forming a tight seal around the areola with the upper and lower lips. Babies thrust their tongues under their mothers' nipple and draw it back into their mouths, while compressing the areola. Rather than sucking, babies really press the milk into their mouths. After each such compression, babies loosen their jaws slightly to allow the pools to refill.

How Much Milk Is Produced? Milk production depends on a number of factors. We've already talked about one important one—demand. The more your baby drinks, the more milk you'll produce and the steadier your supply will become. Babies usually consume about 80% of the milk in your breasts. To further stimulate production, you should hand or pump express the remaining 20%.

An adequate supply of blood is also needed. Your reserves must first serve the vital needs of your body, then that of the alveoli. If an insufficient flow is left for the alveoli, milk production will be reduced. To prevent this, make sure you get plenty of protein, fluids, and calories. (See Chapter 4.)

Probably the biggest factor in let-down failures is the influence of emotions. Your pituitary gland, which signals hormone production, is tied to your hypothalamus—the "emotion" center of your brain. Strong emotional jolts, tension, or anger can stop the hormones' release. This is why relaxation is such an important part of your breastfeeding routine.

Composition of Breast Milk

In Chapter 1, you were told that breast milk is the perfect food for your baby—and it is. No formula can simulate the 100 or more components of breast milk; in fact, researchers are still trying to determine some of their functions. Let's take a closer look at why breast milk is best for your baby.

Colostrum

During the first few days after birth, your breasts produce colostrum. One single feeding of colostrum could increase your baby's immunity to certain infections for up to six months, other factors being favorable. It's that important! Your baby will receive colostrum until your regular milk comes in; your baby's sucking of the colostrum stimulates actual milk production to occur. In comparison to mature breast milk, colostrum has more vitamin A, minerals, and nitrogen, twice as much protein, and less fat and sugar.

Mature Milk

Your first "real" milk will come in approximately five days after birth. Actually, the entire first four weeks is a transition period, with your milk gradually increasing in fat and lactose content and decreasing in protein, sodium, and chloride. After this month period, you'll be producing approximately 1 pint of breast milk daily. This will increase to about a pint and a half by the sixth month, depending on your baby's needs. If you are breastfeeding twins or triplets, which is quite a job, your supply may increase even more significantly.

Mature breast milk contains 20 calories per ounce, though the "hind," or end, milk may contain as many as 35 calories per ounce. Calories are the energy units contained in food. A certain amount of calories are needed daily to maintain growth and good health. Your baby will require close to 50 calories per pound weight daily for normal growth and good health. This means a 6-pound baby would require 300 calories per day. Some babies want more, others want less according to their metabolism, body size, and activity level.

Protein. While we can get protein from meats and a variety of other foods as well, your baby must depend on your milk to meet this daily requirement. For your baby, protein serves as the basic material for cellular growth and repair—plus it is in the most digestible form available. Breast milk has just the right amount of protein for your baby in a form that can be used the most adequately.

Human milk proteins, *lactalbumins*, are digested with almost 100% efficiency because they remain nearly fluid in baby's stomach. Premature babies benefit from breast milk because the proteins contain an amino acid, taurine, which is necessary for proper brain development.

Carbohydrates. The greatest percentage of calories in breast milk comes from carbohydrates which is a very good thing for your baby. One reason why breast milk is so much more efficient is that carbohydrate calories are fast and easy for your baby's system to break down and use for immediate energy. And with all the crying and crawling that lies ahead, your baby will need as much energy as possible.

The main carbohydrate found in breast milk is milk sugar, or *lactose*. Lactose gives your milk a sweet, sugary taste and has the added benefits of making baby's breath more pleasant and stools less odorous. It also creates acidity in baby's stomach, which discourages bacteria. The cow's milk base in some formulas, on the other hand, creates an alkaline environment in the stomach, which promotes the growth of organisms. This is one reason bottlefed babies have more sour smelling bowel movements.

Fats. Fats are likewise needed for energy and as a source of vitamins A, E, and D. Breast milk contains partially saturated fats, while cow's milk and formulas have saturated fats that are difficult for an infant to digest. Along with fats, breast milk has a high level of cholesterol. Babies initially need cholesterol for brain development.

The fat content of your milk is, to say the least, unique; it varies from the beginning to the end of the feeding. The highest level comes at the end of feeding. This arrangement acts as a natural control on overeating, the richer milk filling baby's stomach and stopping your infant's nursing.

Vitamins. The concentration of vitamins in breast milk is optimum for your baby's good health. Rarely will a deficiency occur, but the vitamin content will vary somewhat according to your diet.

There are two types of vitamins, fat-soluble and water-soluble. Fat-soluble vitamins—A, D, E, and K—can be stored in your baby's body and all but D are in some form supplied in breast milk from your own liver and other body stores. At times, vitamin K and vitamin D supplements may be required; your doctor will advise you on this matter. Vitamin K protects your baby against postnatal hemorrhage and is a main factor in proper blood clotting, while vitamin D helps the development of strong bones and teeth.

Water-soluble vitamins, like vitamin C (ascorbic acid) and the B vitamins, must be supplied in your diet. Chapter 4 will tell you which foods are rich in these essential nutrients. If you eat right, your baby should require no supplements.

Minerals. While the mineral content of breast milk is somewhat lower than that of formulas, those minerals present are better utilized. The only mineral supplement which may be needed is fluoride, which is not passed on well from your body.

Iron is the most vital mineral your baby needs to develop. The iron in breast milk is tied to a protein that permits it to be almost completely assimilated into baby's system. Babies over three months, and premature and underweight babies, may require supplemental iron. Again, consult your doctor.

Preparing Your Breasts for Nursing

The best overall preparation for nursing is staying emotionally and physically healthy. Most women have no trouble with their nipples once they begin breastfeeding. However, yours may be particularly sensitive. We at Evenflo recommend that you pay special attention to your breasts at this time to prepare them for your baby's vigorous nursing.

Bathing. During the last trimester, avoid soaps and lotions containing alcohol. Alcohol is extremely drying to your nipples and interferes with the lubrication of the Montgomery's glands. The best thing to do is avoid soaps altogether. Powders, too, can have a drying effect. Just wash your nipples daily with a cloth soaked in clear, warm water. Let air dry completely.

After your bath, briskly but gently rub each nipple with a terry cloth towel to toughen them. Massage can also help: Cup one breast with your hand, press your fingers and thumb together and inward toward your chest wall, circle your breast with a massaging motion, then switch to the other breast and repeat.

Exercise. In general, your baby's frequent nursing will be sufficient to toughen your nipples. However, during pregnancy, exercises, such as nipple rolling and nipple stretching, can help familiarize you with your breasts while toughening them and preventing discomfort. Start at least six weeks before your baby's birth for the maximum benefits.

Nipple Rolling and Stretching. Hold your nipple near its base between the thumb and forefingers of one hand. Slowly pull the nipple outward, turning it up and then down. Do this several times with each nipple until you feel a slight bit of discomfort. It should not be painful. You may want to rub in a breast cream while you exercise to keep your skin supple.

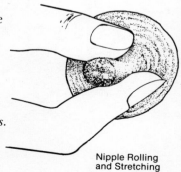

Nipple Rolling
and Stretching

Inverted and Flat Nipples. With an inverted nipple, the tip is flat or appears pushed in, the opposite of its correct

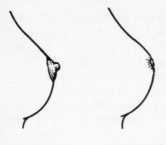

Normal Nipple   Inverted Nipple

shape. Inverted and flat nipples may be somewhat of a problem when nursing, but in most cases they can be corrected through exercise. The Hoffman technique, developed by Dr. J. Brooks Hoffman of Connecticut, was especially designed to draw inverted nipples out to normal.

Draw an imaginary cross on your nipple. Place your thumbs on each end of the horizontal line, locating them directly at the base of the nipple. Press in and at the same time pull the areola away from the nipple. Repeat this five times in this direction; then reposition your thumbs at the top and bottom of the nipple and repeat. Try to practice the Hoffman technique the first thing every morning when you get up. You are loosening the tightness at the base to help the nipple protrude out at a normal position.

Retractile Nipples. These nipples appear normal but may actually be more of a problem than the inverted kind. Retractile nipples are attached to your ribs, so that they pull back when

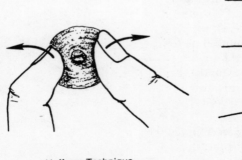

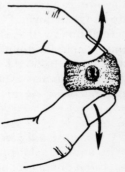

Hoffman Technique

your baby tries to
suck. Try gently
squeezing your
nipple. If it doesn't
project out but
retreats instead, it
may be retractile.
Hoffman exercises
may help
somewhat if
practiced during
pregnancy.
You can also
adjust your

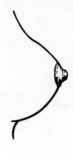

Normal Nipple

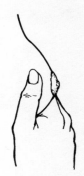

Retractile Nipple

feeding position to bring baby closer to your nipple. (See
Chapter 3.)

Other Helps. Air and the friction created by your clothing
rubbing against your nipples is also beneficial for toughening.
If you can, go without a bra for part of the day. If you feel
uncomfortable without support, either cut the fronts out of a
regular bra or wear a nursing bra with the flaps down. Direct
sunlight, in carefully timed amounts, is also good for toughening and may heal tender areas.

3

Beginning to Nurse

The time has come for all your careful preparations to pay off. You're ready to breastfeed your baby. Breastfeeding is a natural thing and you're going to do just fine. However, it doesn't hurt to practice positive thinking. If you convince yourself that breastfeeding will be a breeze, it more than likely will be!

It is not possible to overly emphasize the importance of relaxation. If you are relaxed during breastfeeding, your baby will also be relaxed. If you are not relaxed, you will not only upset your baby but you will decrease your supply of milk. So relax! Make nursing a soothing time. Listen to some music, find a comfortable nursing position, and remember that breastfeeding gets easier as you go along. Don't let feelings of insecurity rob you and your baby of a rewarding experience.

Getting Baby to Feed

After delivery when your infant is brought to you for the first feeding session, you may notice that baby needs a little coaching in grasping the nipple. You can help baby by either teasing the mouth with your nipple or touching the cheek closest to your breast. Because of an innate rooting reflex, the baby will turn toward the breast. Be careful not to touch both cheeks or shove the breast in your infant's face. You will scare baby and possibly disrupt that feeding session. To ensure that

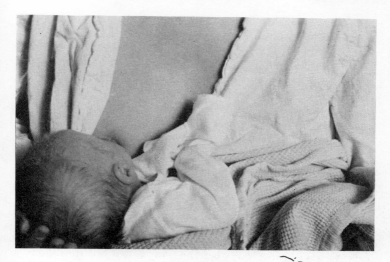

the nipple and areola are in baby's mouth, lift the breast from below. The nipple will be in a position that is easy for baby to grasp. Continue taking baby from your breast until your infant grasps the areola. Help baby along by compressing your nipple and areola between your index and middle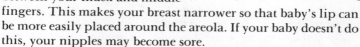
fingers. This makes your breast narrower so that baby's lip can be more easily placed around the areola. If your baby doesn't do this, your nipples may become sore.

Don't be surprised if your baby is not particularly interested in feeding the first few times. Consider these as opportunities for learning and getting to know your baby. After the first few days baby will get down to some serious and enthusiastic suckling. In response to this increase in demand, there will be an increase in the supply of your breast milk.

Your baby may be a natural dawdler or idler. Keep baby's attention by tickling the cheek, teasing the mouth with your nipple (baby recognizes the smell of milk), or talking softly to your child. Remember that breastfeeding is not simply a time to eat. This is the best opportunity that you and your baby have for developing a strong bond.

Keep in mind when feeding that your baby breathes, for the most part, through the nose. Make sure that your breast is not blocking baby's breathing. Simply pressing a finger to the part of the breast closest to the nose usually helps. Some mothers adapt a feeding position that eliminates the problem. The infant's legs are placed under the mother's arms and around her waist. This forces the baby's head away from the breast and allows for easier breathing.

Nursing Positions

You will most likely use the lying down position the first few times you feed your infant. Ask a nurse for assistance. The nurse will either place the baby on your chest or you may lie on your side. Place pillows behind your head and back for support. Place a folded blanket or a thin pillow under the baby. This raises baby's head to a level close to your breast. When it's time to change breasts, place baby on your chest and gently roll over. Cradle your baby with your lowered arm and proceed as before. Cesarean mothers can use this and the other two positions equally as well.

The football hold is another popular position. To feed baby from your right breast settle your child in under your right arm. When your baby finishes nursing on that breast, you can easily switch to the other.

Feeling fitter already? Well celebrate by trying the sitting position. It is the one preferred by most nursing mothers. Find a comfortable chair in which to nurse or try sitting upright in bed. Have a glass of water ready on a nearby table in case you become thirsty. Prop your feet on a stool and relax. If your feet are not properly supported, you may tense your abdominal and pelvic

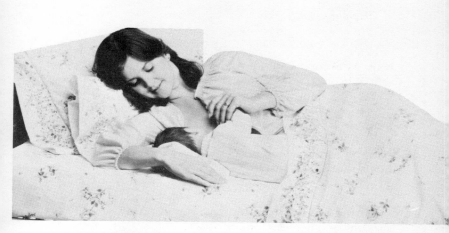

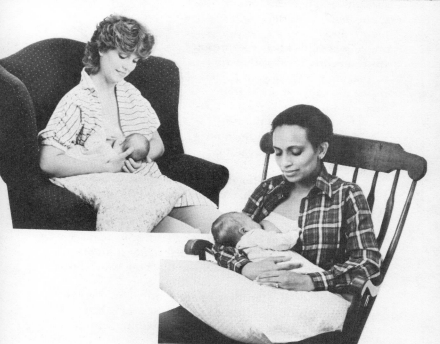

muscles, causing discomfort. Rest the baby crosswise on your body. Your infant's head will probably rest in the crook of your arm. When you want to change breasts, simply break the suction and change baby's position.

It does not matter which nursing position you choose as long as you and your baby are comfortable. Discomfort decreases the let-down reflex. You may find that you prefer using one position for different times of the day. Experiment. You'll eventually find what's best for you.

Breaking the Suction

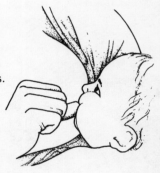

After your baby has finished suckling at one breast, do not immediately pull the infant's mouth away from your nipple and areola. This hurts your nipples. Instead gently break the suction by placing the tip of your finger inside the baby's mouth. Some mothers simply press their breasts away from the baby's mouth, while still others press down on the baby's chin, thus breaking the suction.

Special Positions for Retractile Nipples. When your nipple is attached to your rib, your baby has a difficult time getting it into his mouth at all. Here are two variations that may help.

For the first position, place your baby on a pillow on your lap so that baby is at breast level and both your hands are free. Support the baby's head with your left hand (if nursing on the right side) and keep your breast from blocking baby's breathing with the other.

The second is a variation on the football hold. Again prop your baby on pillows. Use the hand of the arm baby is under to bring the head to breast level and aid breathing with the other.

Burping

Sometimes air is swallowed when your infant is nursing. Although a breastfed infant does not take in as much air as a bottlefed baby, letting what air has been swallowed stay in the stomach can cause discomfort. Burping usually eliminates the chances of your child feeling uncomfortable.

It is necessary for you to burp your baby after the completion of nursing on each breast. By relieving any discomfort felt after nursing on the first breast, you peak your little one's interest in feeding from the second breast. The second burping makes baby comfortable for sleeping or any other activity. Occasionally, burping prior to feeding may also be a good idea in cases where your baby was crying and had swallowed air before being placed to your breast.

There are three standard ways to burp your baby. Each method requires the same necessary accessories. You need either a diaper or a washcloth to protect your clothes from baby's slight spitting up. They also are handy for quick baby cleanups.

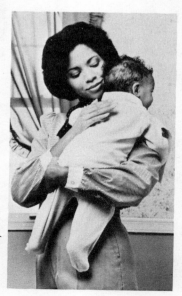

Vertical Position. Hold your baby vertically against your shoulder. Gently rub or pat baby's back. Don't thump or pound! The air won't come up any faster the more enthusiastically you pat.

Sitting Position. You can also have your infant sit on your lap. Support the body with one hand and gently rub the back with your other hand.

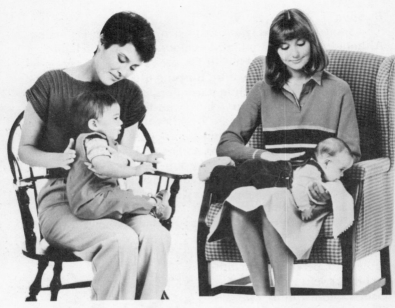

Horizontal Position. Using the third method, place your child stomach-down on your lap, turn the head to one side, then gently rub the back.

My Baby Won't Burp. Don't be surprised if your baby does not burp after every feeding. The amount of air intake differs among all babies. If your child is one of many babies who won't burp, don't continue to pat the back. Simply place baby in the crib, making sure that your child is either on one side or on the stomach. If there is some air itching to get out, you can be sure that it will do so.

Your baby might also be the type that must be burped frequently. That's normal too! Remember to burp your baby as often as needed. Once the air is released, your baby will be more comfortable and will be able to continue to eat because there will be more room in the stomach.

Five Commonly Asked Questions

Especially if this is your first baby, your mind is going to be buzzing with questions. But if you don't come out and ask them, you'll never find out the answers. This may sound like common sense, but many new mothers are afraid that asking too many "what ifs" will make them look silly.

If you can think of a question relating to breastfeeding your baby, it's important enough to ask. Here are some answers to a few common questions.

What if It Hurts?

You are already familiar with the let-down reflex, the brief tingle in your breast felt at the beginning of a nursing session. Also you are aware that during the first few days you may have uterine contractions (which help the uterus return to normal) when you nurse. So in effect you've answered your own question. From what you've already read, you've learned that it is not unusual for most nursing mothers to feel some discomfort when they begin breastfeeding. You as a novice nursing mother are going to have the same experiences. So relax when you feel a twinge. Your body is getting used to having your baby suckling at your breast.

Now and then, a general feeling of discomfort does not go away in a few days. Maybe your nipples have become very sore and cracked. If this is ever the case, contact your doctor or speak with a nurse. They can tell you how to alleviate any soreness. Chapter 7 discusses more fully the types of problems nursing mothers have and what to do to ease any discomfort.

One Breast or Both?

It is best to completely empty one breast and then start on the other if your baby is still hungry. At the next feeding session, offer the second breast first. (Use a safety pin attached to your nursing bra to remind you which breast was last suckled.) By using both breasts for nursing, you ensure that the necessary supply of milk is more easily maintained. Remember the unique supply/demand relationship that exists between the nursing couple.

Try to use both breasts three to five minutes at each feeding the first day. Using both breasts will decrease engorgement and discomfort, making it easier for your baby to nurse. You may be tempted to nurse longer but if you do, your nipples may become sore and tender. Add one or two minutes each time you nurse the second day. Gradually increase the nursing time until you nurse about 10 minutes on the first breast and up to 20 minutes on the second. Don't worry about timing yourself exactly. Your baby can empty your breasts in less than 10 minutes, but may be tired when it's time to nurse on the second one. Also, a baby needs time to just suck, and sucking helps make more breast milk.

Sometimes your baby may be fussy and decide to nurse on one breast only. Try to coax your little one by putting sugar water on the nipple or by always offering that breast first. Eventually baby will give in, but you may have to express milk from that breast in the meantime to maintain your supply.

How Often Should I Feed My Baby?

Your baby may want to nurse anywhere from 6 to 11 times in 24 hours, especially during the first two to four weeks. A general guideline is not to nurse your infant more often than every two hours; however, while young, you should never let baby go more than four to five hours without nursing.

Feeding Schedules. The question of how often to feed easily turns into a lively discussion of the merits of scheduled versus demand feeding. Many parents before you have tried and many after you are going to try to place their babies on strict three- or four-hour nursing schedules. The reasoning behind scheduled feedings seems to stem from a belief that babies benefit best from routines and order. Sounds reasonable, doesn't it? Unfortunately, someone forgot to tell the babies!

Babies have individual schedules. During the first few weeks some babies eat every three hours and some every four. Others want to eat every two hours. If this is the case, don't worry; it doesn't mean that you don't have enough milk. Your baby may simply like to nurse or may feel uncomfortable if taking in more than a small amount at a feeding.

Gradually your baby will get on a schedule that you can more or less depend upon. For the first week or so, you may think that your baby has a bottomless pit for a tummy. But by four months, your infant should be feeding only four or five times daily. This schedule is called self-regulation, or demand feeding.

If your baby cries more often than every two or three hours, hunger may not be the cause. Check the diaper or make sure the baby is not too warm or too cold. Also consider what you may have eaten prior to nursing; some gas-producing foods and liquids containing caffeine can make a baby cranky. If you don't find the reason for baby's crying, just rocking may help.

Modified Demand Schedules. Modified demand borrows the best concepts from scheduled and demand feeding theories. It

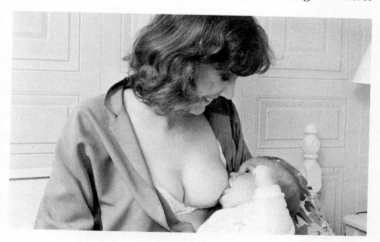

blends the need for a routine that doesn't overly disrupt the needs of other family members with the unique nursing requirements of your child. The result is a flexible feeding schedule to which everyone eventually becomes accustomed.

Is Baby Getting Enough?

As long as your baby is satisfied between feedings, sleeping well, gaining weight, and has approximately six wet (not just damp) diapers a day, don't worry. Your child is getting enough breast milk on which to thrive. Remember that breastfed babies may not gain weight as quickly as bottlefed babies. This is perfectly all right.

Around six weeks and again at three months, your baby may seem to be hungrier and want to nurse more often than usual. Additional suckling will produce more milk, so nurse more frequently if that's what baby wants.

Once in a while a doctor informs a nursing mother that she has insufficient breast milk. This conclusion is the result of the physician's evaluation of baby's physical development. When your child doesn't gain enough weight, supplemental bottles may be necessary . If this occurs while you are breastfeeding, don't give up. It's not as final as it sounds. Before you begin to give supplementary bottles to your baby, try increasing your milk supply by following some of these suggestions.

First, remember the importance of relaxation and self-confidence. Many nursing mothers have allowed nervousness and a lack of confidence in themselves to put a stop to nursing. Realize that you're both new at this. You can't expect everything to be perfect at the beginning. Keeping this in mind helps you regain any sudden drops in your supply of milk.

Second, try to increase the number of feeding sessions between you and your baby. You're probably getting tired of reading this, but it's true—the more baby nurses, the more milk comes in.

Some mothers have successfully increased their milk supplies by expressing milk. The principle underlying this suggestion is similar to the one behind increasing nursing sessions. The breasts are stimulated more often; therefore, the milk supply is increased.

Finally, check to make sure that you are taking good care of yourself. We cannot say enough about the importance of rest. If you've been overdoing it, slow down. Having lots of visitors and being too active aren't helping you or your baby. Also try to maintain a healthy diet. Eat the correct selection of foods from the four food groups, drink plenty of liquids (which is vitally important), and ask your doctor about taking vitamin supplements. You don't have to eat a lot; just make every calorie count. See the following chapter for a more detailed discussion of taking care of yourself.

What about Overfeeding?

Breastfed babies rarely, if ever, overfeed. They know how much they need. So don't worry that your baby is getting too much milk. The only time overfeeding may be a possibility is if your breastfed baby spits up or regurgitates a lot. In this case, reduce your baby's time at the breast and note what happens. If the problem continues, consult your baby's doctor.

Hospital Routines

The earlier you touch, feel, and handle your new baby, the better it is for you, your husband, and your newborn. The very first hours of life are usually best, even right in the delivery room. So ask to have your baby placed at your breast immediately after delivery. If that is not possible, most hospitals will bring your baby to you within the first 4 to 12 hours after birth. In some communities if the mother prefers, she and the baby can stay together in the same room. This advancement in family-oriented childbirth is called rooming-in.

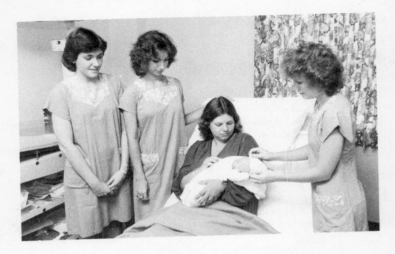

Rooming-in. This type of hospital stay permits easy scheduling of breastfeeding sessions. Whenever your baby is hungry, you are right there, ready to satisfy the hunger pangs. Nurses are available to help you with all aspects of care and feeding. Visitation rules for those other than your husband may be restrictive, but the benefits to your new family outweigh the lack of visitors. If you do not feel comfortable about immediately caring for your baby around the clock, consider modified rooming-in. This permits you to have the baby with you during the day. At night the nurses return the baby to the nursery and bring your newborn to your room only when hungry.

Special Births

Many people harbor misconceptions about what type of childbirth procedures permit breastfeeding and which babies can successfully breastfeed. They believe that only babies delivered vaginally are capable of breastfeeding. This is not true.

Cesarean Sections

If you are like many new mothers, you may have had your baby by a cesarean. But this is no reason to prevent you from breastfeeding. In fact, it may provide a better reason for you to try nursing your baby. Though cesareans are quite a natural thing these days, you may still feel deprived because you weren't actually able to experience birth. The important thing, however, is that your baby is healthy—and breastfeeding can help keep baby that way.

How soon breastfeeding begins depends upon you and your baby. Assuming that the birth was routine and you carried the baby to full-term, breastfeeding can begin as soon as the anesthesia wears off. You may begin to nurse right in the delivery room or recovery room if a spinal or epidural anesthetic was used. In cases when general anesthetic is used, you should be able to nurse as soon as you and the baby are completely alert. To keep you both comfortable, have a nurse elevate your head and legs and place your baby on a pillow.

Premature Delivery

The question is not whether or not a premature infant *can* breastfeed, but how soon breastfeeding can begin. Many experts have found that mother's milk is best for the premature baby.

As long as your premature infant is strong enough to suckle at your breast, breastfeeding is possible. This depends upon baby's condition and development at birth. Even when a baby is too small or too weak to nurse, breast milk can still provide its benefits. While baby is still in the nursery, the nurses will feed your expressed milk to the infant through a tube or a special nipple. When conditions improve, you may even be able to feed baby yourself. Not only will your newborn benefit from your milk, but baby will also benefit from all your love.

Some mothers continue to express milk when they leave the hospital even when their babies must remain in the nursery.

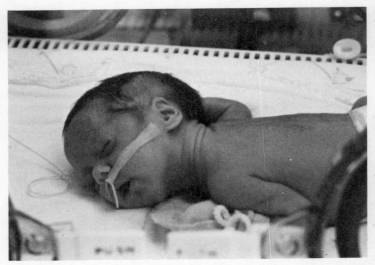

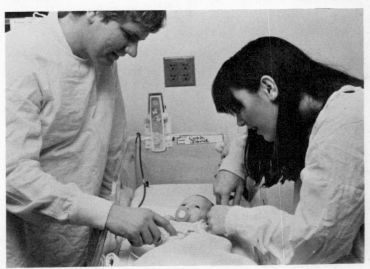

46

This expressed milk can be frozen, saved, and used later for supplemental feedings. Plus, expressing now prepares them for breastfeeding once their babies are home.

Other mothers simply come to the hospital several times a day to actually breastfeed their convalescing babies. (Naturally this will depend on how close the hospital is to your home.) If your infant has become used to a bottle while in the hospital, settling into a breastfeeding routine will take time. Don't worry; baby will eventually and successfully learn to breastfeed.

Multiple Births

Many mothers who give birth to more than one baby during a pregnancy successfully breastfeed with slight modifications.

Twins. You can nurse both twins at once or feed one at a time. Feeding both at once is preferable. It saves time and may even keep both babies on the same schedule. Whatever you do decide, remember to offer alternating breasts to your twins. Each breast has its own supply and each twin makes varying demands on it. Alternating ensures an adequate supply.

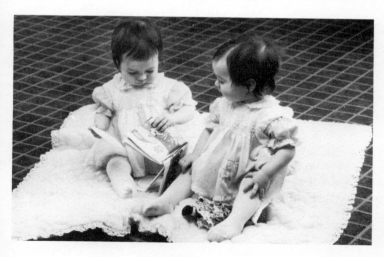

It is also important for you to try other means of keeping up your supply of milk. So attempt to express your milk between breastfeeding sessions, every three hours if your twins are premature. This not only increases your milk supply, but it also provides you with much needed supplemental bottles (for those times when you don't have the time to nurse).

Standard nursing positions also need adjustments. Read the section on comfortable positions; then experiment to find what's most comfortable for you.

Finally, speak with other mothers of twins who have successfully breastfed. There's nothing comparable to talking with someone who has already experienced what you are now living. Veteran nursing mothers have a treasure of helpful hints that they are only too willing to share. So enjoy! Nursing twins is "twice" as rewarding.

Three or More. If you have more than two infants, you can still breastfeed them. It may take a little longer, but it definitely is more convenient than bottlefeeding. Many of the suggestions for nursing twins are also applicable for three or more. The biggest difference comes at feeding time. There is no way that all of your babies can nurse during one feeding session. You are going to have to alternate which babies are breastfed and which are bottlefed. It takes some scheduling, but it all works out. You may not be able to breastfeed for many months; however, that is not what is important. Your babies benefit from any amount of time spent suckling at your breast.

From Hospital to Home

Home, sweet, home—well, sort of. Life at home with a new baby isn't going to be quite like it used to be. Babies enjoy being a challenge—one you'll eventually get used to. Meanwhile just think, you won't have to worry about how to spend a boring evening any more; you won't have any!

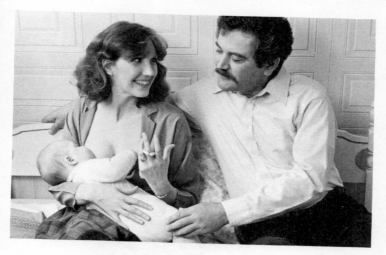

You may also feel that all of you are on the baby's schedule, which normally isn't a bad idea except that it always seems to be changing! Again, don't worry. Just as you modified your infant's feeding schedule, you can adapt the day-to-day schedule. All you need is a lot of patience and more than your fair share of flexibility. Remember that you've learned a great deal in the hospital, possibly more than you realize. You'll eventually settle down and be able to put all of this newfound learning to use.

Once you've worked out a compromise schedule between yourself and your baby, you only have three other feeding hurdles with which to deal. They are night feedings, supplemental feedings, and weaning. This section discusses the first two. Chapter 8 covers everything you need to know about weaning.

Night Feedings

Some mothers enjoy night feedings. They welcome the special warmth and coziness that late night nursings bring. Whether mother and baby nurse in the warmth of a bed or snuggle together under a comforter on a sofa, this feeding is always comforting and relaxing.

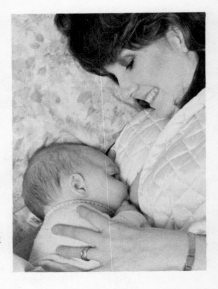

Other mothers can never adjust themselves to midnight or 2:00 *a.m.* feedings. They hear baby fussing and know that hunger cries are not far away. Nevertheless, they are not discouraged. They realize that as baby grows older, the night feedings will stop.

Right at this moment you probably don't know what your attitude to night feedings is. Whatever you decide, you must remember not to try to break your child's late night feeding routine. If you are following the demand or self-regulating schedule, and even if you have baby on a strict schedule, you know that your baby needs these feedings. When ready, baby will forget all about nighttime feedings and sleep through the night.

When Do Night Feedings End? The cessation of night feedings is an individual characteristic of every baby. Some infants begin sleeping through the night as early as one month; others have been known to require night feedings until 12 to 18 months. So while you're waiting for your baby to reach that developmental benchmark, make your night feedings easier by maintaining a relaxed and comfortable attitude.

Supplemental Feedings

If you are not producing enough milk for your baby to consume and you and your doctor have done everything possible to increase your milk supply, supplemental bottles are a must. If, however, you only want to substitute bottles for breastfed sessions, do not do so until lactation is well established. When you switch to supplementary bottles earlier than one month, baby has a more difficult time readjusting to suckling from a human nipple. Why? Because it is easier to get milk from the nipple of a bottle than it is to get it from your nipple.

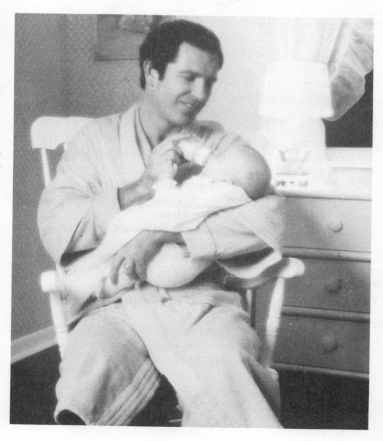

Helpful Hints. Try to give only supplemental bottles that contain expressed milk. Babies accept bottles of breast milk more readily than those filled with formula or cow's milk because they're familiar with the taste. So don't be surprised if baby balks when given a bottle of anything else.

Some nursing mothers have also found that their babies won't take a bottle from them; however, they will do so from someone with whom they do not associate breastfeeding. This is an excellent opportunity for a father to become more involved in feeding sessions and nurturing. He may want to take the late night or early morning feedings to give you an uninterrupted six to eight hours of sleep.

Finally, remember to still cuddle your baby even when you give a bottle. Don't just prop the bottle in baby's mouth. You may not be able to breastfeed, but you can still hold your child close and give your love.

Vitamins. We know from Chapter 2 that your baby gets the necessary supply of various vitamins and minerals by breastfeeding. They are all inherent in your milk. However, vitamin D and fluoride aren't received through nursing. Many doctors recommend giving breastfed babies supplements of these beginning approximately three weeks after birth.

Vitamin D, the sunshine vitamin, is especially important. By absorbing calcium and phosphates, it makes itself a necessary ingredient for healthy bone and tooth development. Because breast milk has only traces of vitamin D, specially-developed infant drops are required.

Healthy babies also require fluoride supplements, especially if the water in their communities is not fluoridated. Researchers have discovered that your baby's teeth begin to form early in pregnancy. The minerals, vitamins, and other nutrients a baby needs for teeth formation are supplied by the foods you eat. Once born, your infant no longer receives fluoride from you, so drops are recommended during infancy to protect against cavities.

What's Ahead

You've got your baby off to a good start breastfeeding. But what about you? Take a look in the mirror. Are you getting nasty rings under your eyes? Are those quick meals of a candy bar and a soda doing you any good? If you're going to continue breastfeeding successfully, you must take care of yourself. See Chapter 4 for the tips you'll need to know.

4

The Number One Priority—
Take Care of Yourself

Naturally you are concerned with your baby's health, but at the same time you can't afford to forsake your own well-being. If you are undernourished or teetering at the brink of exhaustion, your baby and the rest of your family will also feel the ill effects in one way or another. You've just completed nine months of tiring pregnancy and your body needs time to recuperate and replenish its stores. So for the first few weeks, make an attempt to pamper yourself as much as possible. Forget about the housework and the fuzz balls gathering under the couch. Put caring for your family—and yourself—first. And don't say "No" to help offered by your husband or older children. Even a simple thing such as being brought a glass of water can be a tremendous lift when you are trying to devote your strength to breastfeeding your baby. This is one time when idleness will be rewarded—with a healthy, happy family.

A Diet to Meet Body Needs

The diet you follow should not only help you breastfeed successfully, but should be a step toward better nutrition all life long. Plus, your program can benefit the entire family, helping them attain good nutrition as well.

There's nothing really "special" about the diet you should follow while breastfeeding; try "sensible" instead. You need a well-balanced, varied diet that encompasses the four basic food groups: meats and proteins, fruits and vegetables, breads and

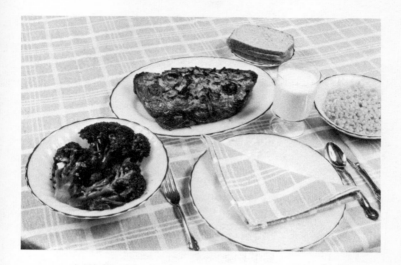

cereals, and milk and milk products. And while your doctor may prescribe vitamin or mineral supplements, these in no way replace the essential nutrients—and calories—you receive from the food you eat.

How Many Calories Do I Need?

As discussed in Chapter 1, breastfeeding doesn't mean that you have to eat for two. You'll need approximately 500 to 1,000 more calories daily than your normal intake, most of which will be burned up in milk production. While breastfeeding, you may find that your appetite initially increases. However, this will subside as you begin to wean your baby onto other foods.

If you are undernourished, you'll feel the effects before your baby. Remember the old saying "You lose a tooth for every baby"? What it really means is that needed nutrients, such as calcium, will be robbed from your own stores to provide for your baby. With the deficiencies already present from the strains of pregnancy and labor, any further depletion could be serious.

Your husband can help by making sure that you take the time out to eat right, even if it means hiding the candy jar on the top shelf out of your reach. The nutritional quality of the food is sometimes more important than the quantity. Try to get into the habit of eating breakfast, as well as lunch and dinner. The morning is when you'll need the most energy and baby will be feeding the most heavily. When eating, take your time and chew your food to aid digestion. If you find you can't eat enough in three meals, try eating several smaller meals instead.

What Should I Eat?

Your doctor will probably prescribe a diet for you while you're breastfeeding. It should be high in proteins and contain a minimum of starches, fatty foods, and sweets. In general, you should eat the required number of servings.

Basic Food Group Requirements	
Group	Servings
Meats and Proteins	4
Milk and Milk Products	5
Breads and Cereals	4
Fruits and Vegetables	
Vitamin C rich fruits and vegetables	1
Dark green vegetables	1
Other fruits and vegetables	1

Source—U.S. Dept. of Health and Human Services pamphlet, *Breast Feeding*.

In addition, you'll need about 2 tablespoons of fats and oils. Some junk foods are all right, but don't fill up on them in place of necessary foods. Switch to nutritious snacks such as fruits, raw vegetables, and cheese.

Meats and Proteins. Both animal and vegetable sources provide protein as well as B vitamins and iron. Protein permits growth; it is broken down into amino acids which are absorbed into the bloodstream and are used by your baby's body to build new cells. B vitamins are essential for obtaining energy from

Meats and Proteins	
Choices	Per Serving
Animal protein	
Beef (ground, cube, roast, or chop)	2–3 oz (56–84 gm)
Clams	4 large or 9 small
Eggs	2 medium
Fish (fillet or steak)	2 oz
Fish sticks	3 sticks
Frankfurters	2
Lamb (ground, cube, roast, or chop)	2–3 oz
Luncheon meat	3 slices
Organ meats: heart, kidney, liver, or tongue	2–3 oz
Oysters	8–12 medium
Pork, ham (ground, roast, or chop)	2–3 oz
Poultry: chicken, duck, or turkey	2–3 oz
Rabbit	2–3 oz
Sausage links	4 links
Shellfish: crab, lobster, scallops, or shrimp	2–3 oz
Spareribs	6 medium ribs
Tuna fish	2–3 oz
Veal (ground, cube, roast, or chop)	2–3 oz
Vegetable protein	
Canned beans: garbanzo, kidney, lima, or pork and beans	1 cup (240 ml)
Dried beans and peas	1 cup
Nut butters: cashew butter, peanut butter, etc.	1/4 cup
Nuts	1/2 cup (120 ml)
Sunflower seeds	1/2 cup
Tofu (soybean curd)	1 cup

Source—U.S. Dept. of Health and Human Services pamphlet, *Breast Feeding*.

food while iron is needed for the formation of red blood cells. Iron is also a must for your body to replenish its supplies. By choosing a variety of animal and vegetable proteins each day, for example two of each, you will easily meet your daily protein requirements. A lactating woman needs more protein than would be normal and a fair amount more than her husband.

Milk and Milk Products. Milk and milk products are the best sources of calcium, which builds strong bones and teeth and helps your baby's body convert soft cartilage into bone. It also makes for healthy nerves and muscles. Dairy products also contain protein, several B vitamins, and vitamins A and D. Vitamin A is needed for growth and good vision, plus it protects your baby from infection. Vitamin D enables your baby to use calcium. Your doctor may recommend a calcium supplement if you don't like milk or are allergic to it. However, calcium tablets may be less readily adsorbed into your bloodstream.

Milk and Milk Products	
Choices*	**Per Serving**
Cheese (except Camembert or cream)	1 slice (1-1/2 oz or 42 gm)
Cheese spread	4 tbsps (60 ml)
Cocoa (made with milk)	1-1/4 cups (10 oz or 300 ml)
Cottage cheese	1-1/3 cups (320 ml)
Custard (flan)	1 cup (240 ml)
Ice cream	1-1/2 cups (360 ml)
Milk	
buttermilk	1 cup
chocolate (made with whole or nonfat milk)	1-1/4 cups
evaporated	1/2 cup (4 oz or 120 ml)
goat	1 cup
low-fat	1 cup
nonfat	1 cup
nonfat milk (made from 1/3 cup dry milk powder)	1 cup
nonfat dry milk powder (used in other recipes)	1/3 cup (80 ml)
whole	1 cup
Milk shake	1 cup
Pudding	1 cup
Soup (made with milk)	1-1/2 cups (12 oz or 360 ml)
Yogurt	1 cup

*Not all milk and milk products contain vitamins A and D, so check the label before purchasing.
Source—U.S. Dept. of Health and Human Services pamphlet, *Breast Feeding.*

Breads and Cereals. Breads and cereals have many vital nutrients including iron, phosphorus, zinc, and B vitamins. Whole-grain breads and grain products contain more vitamins

Breads and Cereals	
Choices	**Per Serving**
Whole Grain Products*	
Bread: cracked, whole wheat, or rye	1 slice
Cereal, hot: oatmeal (rolled oats), rolled wheat, cracked wheat, wheat, and malted barley	1/2 cup, cooked (120 ml)
Cereal, ready-to-eat: puffed oats, shredded wheat, wheat flakes, or granola	3/4 cup (180 ml)
Rice, brown	1/2 cup, cooked
Wheat germ	1 tbsp
Enriched Grain Products†	
Bagel	1 small
Bread (all except those listed previously)	1 slice
Cereal, hot: cream of wheat, cream of rice, farina, cornmeal, or grits	1/2 cup, cooked
Cereal, ready-to-eat: (all except those previously mentioned)	3/4 cup (180 ml)
Crackers	4
Macaroni, noodles, or spaghetti	1/2 cup, cooked
Pancake, waffle	1 medium (5″ or 13 cm diameter)
Rice, white	1/2 cup, cooked
Roll, biscuit, muffin, or dumpling	1
Tortilla	1 (6″ or 15 cm diameter)

*Some supermarkets and stores also carry whole wheat macaroni, spaghetti, noodles, tortillas, and pita bread.

†Doughnuts, cakes, pies, and cookies have not been included because they contain mostly calories and very few vitamins and minerals.

Source—U.S. Dept. of Health and Human Services pamphlet, *Breast Feeding.*

and minerals than those that are merely enriched. Enriched grains have one-third of the iron, B vitamins, and niacin removed during refining and then replaced; however, other nutrients, such as calcium, potassium, and magnesium, are lessened considerably during the process. Whole-grain products also give you fiber. Fiber aids your digestive system and may prevent constipation, a common postpartum problem.

Vitamin C Rich Fruits and Vegetables. A particular group of fruits and vegetables contains vitamin C, or ascorbic acid.

Vitamin C Rich Fruits and Vegetables	
Choices	**Per Serving**
Fruits	
Cantaloupe	1/2 medium
Grapefruit	1/2 large
Guava	1/2 small
Mango	1 medium
Orange	1 medium
Papaya	1/2 small
Strawberries	3/4 cup (180 ml)
Tangerine	2 large
Juices (with vitamin C added)	
Grapefruit	1/2 cup (4 oz or 120 ml)
Orange	1/2 cup
Pineapple	1-1/2 cups (12 oz or 360 ml)
Tomato	1-1/2 cups
Vegetables	
Broccoli	1 stalk
Brussels sprouts	3–4
Cabbage	3/4 cup
Cauliflower	3/4 cup
Chili peppers, red or green	1/4 cup (60 ml)
Greens: collard, kale, mustard, or turnip	3/4 cup
Peppers, red or green	1/2 medium
Potato	1 medium
Tomatoes	2 medium
Watercress	3/4 cup

Source—U.S. Dept. of Health and Human Services pamphlet, *Breast Feeding.*

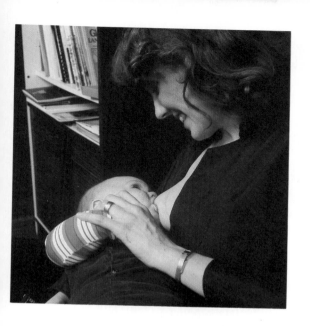

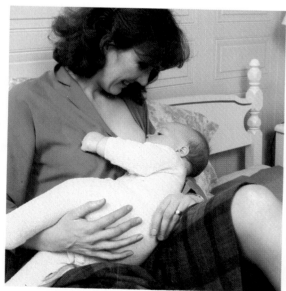

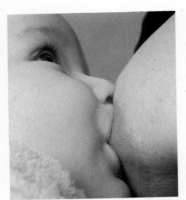

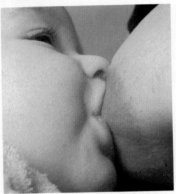

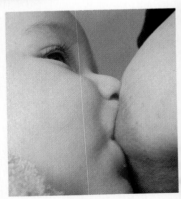

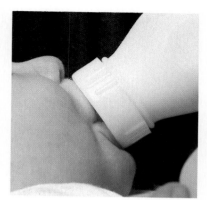

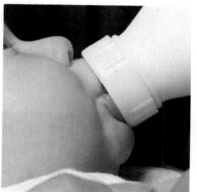

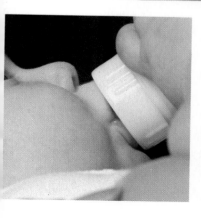

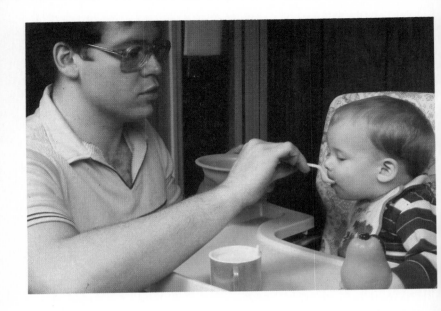

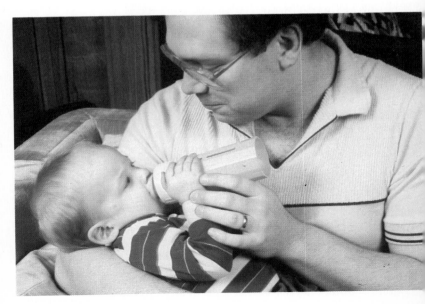

Vitamin C holds body cells together, strengthens blood vessels, promotes healthy gums, and aids in the healing of wounds.

Dark Green Vegetables. Such vegetables are excellent sources of vitamin A and folic acid. Your baby requires vitamin A for bone and tooth formation, good vision, and resistance to infections. Folic acid, a B vitamin, is integral for the formation of blood and other body cells. Because cooking temperatures destroy folic acid, try to eat your dark green vegetables raw whenever possible.

Dark Green Vegetables	
Choices	**Per Serving**
Asparagus	1 cup, raw (240 ml) or 3/4 cup, cooked (180 ml)
Chicory	1 cup, raw or 3/4 cup, cooked
Endive	1 cup, raw or 3/4 cup, cooked
Escarole	1 cup, raw or 3/4 cup, cooked
Greens: beet, collard, kale, mústard, or turnip	1 cup, raw or 3/4 cup, cooked
Lettuce: dark leafy, red leaf, or romaine	1 cup, raw or 3/4 cup, cooked
Scallions	1 cup, raw or 3/4 cup, cooked
Spinach	1 cup, raw or 3/4 cup, cooked

Source—U.S. Dept. of Health and Human Services pamphlet, *Breast Feeding*.

Other Fruits and Vegetables. You should have at least one serving from the "other fruits and vegetables" category each day to supplement your lactation diet plan. Dark yellow fruits and vegetables are excellent sources of vitamin A. These include the following: apricots, persimmons, pumpkin, carrots, sweet potatoes, yams, and winter squash. Like whole-grain products, many are also rich in fiber, which will help regulate your bowel movements. Dried and raw fruits and vegetables are higher in fiber than cooked or canned ones.

Need for Liquids

Because you are using fluids when you produce milk, breastfeeding may leave you feeling dry or parched. To correct

Other Fruits and Vegetables

Choices	Per Serving
Fruits	
Apple	1 medium
Apricot	2 medium
Banana	1 small
Berries	1 cup (240 ml)
Cherries	1/2 cup (120 ml)
Dates	5
Figs	2 large
Fruit cocktail	1/2 cup
Grapes	1/2 cup
Kumquats	3
Nectarines	2 medium
Peach	1 medium
Pear	1 medium
Persimmon	1 small
Pineapple	1/2 cup
Plums	2 medium
Prunes	4 medium
Pumpkin	1/4 cup (60 ml)
Raisins	1/2 cup
Watermelon	1/2 cup
Vegetables	
Artichoke	1 medium
Bamboo shoots	1/2 cup
Beans, green or wax	1/2 cup
Bean sprouts	1/2 cup
Beets	1/2 cup
Carrots	1/2 cup
Cauliflower	1/2 cup
Celery	1/2 cup
Corn	1/2 cup
Cucumber	1/2 cup
Eggplant	1/2 cup
Hominy	1/2 cup
Lettuce: head, Boston, or bibb	1/2 cup
Mushrooms	1/2 cup
Onions	1/2 cup
Parsnips	1/2 cup
Pea pods	1/2 cup

Other Fruits and Vegetables (Cont'd)	
Choices	**Per Serving**
Vegetables (Cont'd)	
Peas	1/2 cup
Radishes	1/2 cup
Sweet potatoes	1 medium
Winter squash	1/2 cup
Yams	1 medium
Zucchini	1/2 cup

Source—U.S. Dept. of Health and Human Services pamphlet, *Breast Feeding.*

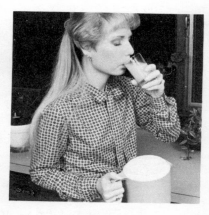

this and prevent constipation, make sure you drink between 8 to 10 glasses of liquid daily. You'll find your quota easier to meet if you have a drink before each nursing session.

Must you drink milk? Not necessarily, although milk is a good source of calcium. You'll have to make up for it by eating more of the other dairy products or taking calcium tablets. Water, drinks without caffeine, or real fruit juices can all supply the fluid you require. Soups also provide some liquid, though often not enough to be significant. With soft drinks, you encounter the opposite problem; they supply the fluid you need but have little or no nutritional value.

For an occasional treat and to break up the monotony, dim the lights and pour a glass of wine for you and your husband during one of the evening feedings. It's a great way to ease tensions and serves to rekindle some of those quiet, romantic moments.

No Time for Diets. Although you may be concerned about returning to your pre-pregnancy weight, this is no time to diet. Fad diets and diet pills can be harmful and do not furnish the nutrients your body needs to continue producing milk. When you use diet aids, you are trying to trick your stomach into believing that it is full and satisfied. You may feel full but may actually be undernourished, especially when you are devoting a good percentage of your caloric intake to lactation and nursing.

Your added weight was gained over a span of nine months; you can't expect it to disappear overnight. Many women leave the delivery room and imagine that they will be able to look in a mirror and see their body back to normal. Unfortunately this is not the case, because the baby and surrounding fluids only account for part of the increase. Breastfeeding, however, will aid you in burning up many of the remaining pounds as long as you don't actually "try to eat for two." By the time your baby is weaned and nearly a year old, your figure should be nearly back to normal.

Vegetarianism. If you have been a vegetarian, it should not have any ill effects on your baby or your breastfeeding ability as long as your diet contains some form of protein—the proper mix of vegetable proteins and sources of vitamin B-12. Fish, chicken, eggs, nuts, and beans are all nonmeat sources that can be incorporated into your vegetarian meal plans. However, if you do not eat any animal proteins, your doctor may have to add a vitamin B-12 supplement to your diet to prevent you or your baby from developing anemia. A vitamin B-12 deficiency can also affect your heart and brain. Also be wary of macrobiotic diets (those consisting basically of whole grains). They are often too limited to allow for adequate nutrition.

Can What I Eat Affect My Baby?

Essentially, everything you eat passes into your milk supply within four to six hours after you ingest it. However, it's rare for any foods to really harm your nursing baby—with the exception of drugs and other substances such as caffeine and nicotine. (See Chapter 5.)

If your baby does seem unusually upset or fussy after a feeding or develops a rash or diarrhea, first look for outside causes of the problem. Did you add any vitamin supplements or switch detergent? If nothing unusual turns up, start eliminating a different food each week from your diet. Concentrate on foods to which you or your husband may be allergic or on those which you may have eaten in unusually large quantities. In some instances, it's a question of "how much" rather than "what" you eat. Problems commonly are caused by milk, citrus fruits, chocolate, and nuts. Cabbage, broccoli, and brussels sprouts may cause gas, and garlic and onions can flavor your milk. Try not to overdo on any of these items.

Exercise Is Excellent

If you really feel the need to lose weight, try exercise rather than a diet. You may discover that all your body was crying out for was a little toning up and tucking in! In fact you really should exercise after a pregnancy because the longer you allow your body to atrophy, the more time it will take for you to get back in shape. Exercise also has the added benefits of reducing tension and irritability and warding off the fatigues of parenthood. And contrary to the old wives' tale, rocking or bouncing around while nursing will not shake up your milk!

When should you start exercising? If you feel up to it, begin your recovery program by taking walks in the hospital. However, avoid stairs until you are more sure of your balance. Remember that your body posture altered during pregnancy to give extra support to your extended abdomen area. Now that the baby is born, your body must again readjust and may make your balance shaky. If you've had a cesarean or any other complications during the birth of your baby, talk to your doctor before starting any potentially harmful overexertion.

Starting Out

While your whole body will need toning, the two main areas requiring attention are your abdomen and pelvic floor. These have been stretched the most during pregnancy and labor and will take the most effort on your part to restore. Afterward, it's on to all the rest. You'll find a thorough postpartum exercise program included in *The Evenflo Guide to A Healthy Pregnancy*.

Abdominal Wall

Supports Internal Organs

The Abdomen. During pregnancy, the muscles of your abdominal wall virtually have doubled in length. Though they will never contract completely back to normal, proper exercise will restore them as much as possible. Refer to a good exercise book for specific exercises such as sit-ups, camel walks, and bridging.

Pelvic Floor. The pelvic floor is the muscle that supports your entire pelvic area. The stretching it undergoes during labor may result in loss of control of your sphincter (anal) muscles as well as those of your vagina. Vaginal contractions and pelvic tilts are particularly good exercises for this region.

Rules for Exercising

Before you jump headfirst into a strenuous exercise program, wait until you have your postpartum doctor's examination. This will give you the peace of mind that you're on the road to recovery and may make you aware of any problem areas that exist. When exercising, begin slowly. Exercise often and for short periods; never overexert yourself to the point of pain. Teeth-gritting is not the point of exercising; however, gradually developing a better, healthier body is. Should you feel nauseated or experience sharp pains, stop immediately and see your doctor.

Rest

Though it's come up many times before in this book, your need for rest can't be overemphasized. True, women do recover from childbirth at widely varying rates. But you don't want to increase the possibility of a long period of recovery if you can help it. The more work and strain you subject your body to during the first few weeks after birth, the longer your recuperation will take. So don't overdo. And try to employ some of the following suggestions.

Get Help

Don't be afraid to admit that you need help, particularly with housework or meal preparation. You'll need to conserve the bulk of your strength just to take care of and breastfeed your baby. Your husband can contribute in many ways: doing chores, going to the store, preparing meals, and taking charge of other children in your family. Even his simple words of encouragement can boost your spirits and soothe your frazzled nerves.

If your husband can't be away from work, ask a relative or close friend to stay over or drop in for the first few days you are home. Besides helping around the house, this person may be able to answer any questions you might have about taking care of the baby—before you reach the point of panic!

Take Time Out

Try to rest as much at home as you did while in the hospital, or at least make a reasonable attempt to do so. Pamper yourself by spending your first three days at home in bed. Remember, you don't become a mother every day! Naps are

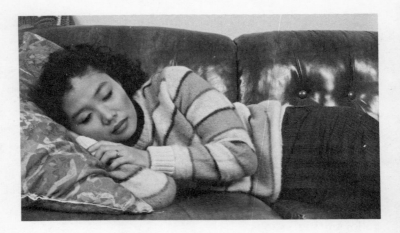

equally important. Try to take one whenever your baby falls asleep or if your husband is home to take charge. You may find that getting eight hours of uninterrupted sleep at night is next to impossible.

Another time you need to be rested and relaxed is right before breastfeeding. If you are calm, your let-down reflex will function more quickly. Sit back in a comfortable chair and close your eyes for five minutes or so before each feeding.

A houseful of relatives and well-wishers is something else you don't need—at least for the first two weeks. Although you may enjoy seeing them, guests unconsciously expect to be entertained. By the time they're on their way out the door, you'll have no energy left to care for your baby.

Sex. Returning to a well-adjusted, regular sex life will also relieve tensions for both of you. (Be sure you get your doctor's okay at a postpartum checkup before resuming.) It's not true that your sex drive will lessen during lactation; however, you may feel unattractive or nervous at the prospect. If your husband doesn't approach you, make the first move yourself. He might be afraid of hurting you or think that you're too wrapped up with the baby to be interested. Start out gently and use a lubricant to alleviate any dryness and to reduce strain on healing areas. Even a little cuddling can help put the frustrations of a long day behind you. Be prepared for interruptions. Your baby doesn't know yet what "do not disturb" really means!

Breast Care While Nursing

As you become increasingly involved with your baby's world, you may start skimping on breast care. But this is just as important now as it was when you were pregnant. If you have sensitive skin, your nipples may become overly dry or cracked. We want to help you prevent this.

Before nursing, wipe your nipples with a cotton ball, rather than a washcloth, dipped in warm water. Washcloths may be too tough on your nipples at this point. Make sure to wash off any lubricants you may have used. It's a good idea to get into the habit of washing your hands before handling your breasts to keep them as clean as possible. After feeding, again wipe your

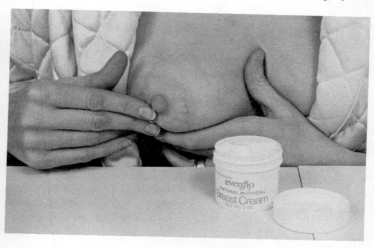

nipples and allow them to air dry for 15 minutes if possible. Rubbing on a breast cream after cleansing will reduce any chafing or discomfort.

Nursing Bras

A good nursing bra can improve your circulation, keep you feeling comfortable, and improve the line of your clothes. You'll need several such bras during nursing to allow for washing and a daily change—or more depending on the extent of leakage you experience. For your own comfort, you may also want to wear your bra while sleeping.

What to Look for in a Bra. Before anything else, a nursing bra must fit. Another style may be more attractive, but if it binds, you could develop plugged ducts.

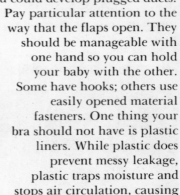

Pay particular attention to the way that the flaps open. They should be manageable with one hand so you can hold your baby with the other. Some have hooks; others use easily opened material fasteners. One thing your bra should not have is plastic liners. While plastic does prevent messy leakage, plastic traps moisture and stops air circulation, causing chafing, cracking, and soreness. Disposable nursing pads that fit inside your bra are a much better alternative. Look for pads made of soft, absorbent fibers that pull moisture away from your skin. This point also applies to the bra itself. Bras with a high percentage of cotton will absorb moisture better and allow your breasts to breathe. Select one with strong, wide, nonelastic straps that provide support without sagging. Your nipples should be held at a position midway between your shoulders and your elbows.

Selecting the Proper Bra Size. The size you are in your eighth month will be close to your breastfeeding bra size, though your breasts may initially become somewhat fuller when your milk comes in. For the correct chest measurement, measure the distance around your back and under your arms and breasts. The cup size is your actual bust measurement (across your back and over your nipples) minus your chest measurement. A 1″ difference is an "A" cup; 2″, a "B" cup, and so on. For example, if your bust measurement is 39″ and your chest measurement is 36″, you'd buy a size 36 bra with a C cup.

Dressing for Breastfeeding

If you are all bundled up in the "layered look" with seven or eight shirts and sweaters, your baby could starve before you could get ready. Some stylish fashions make getting undressed similar to trying to slip out of a straightjacket. Our advice? When you're breastfeeding, stick to comfortable, convenient clothes. Separates, like slacks and sweaters or skirts and blouses, are probably the easiest to work around. Cardigans and pullover

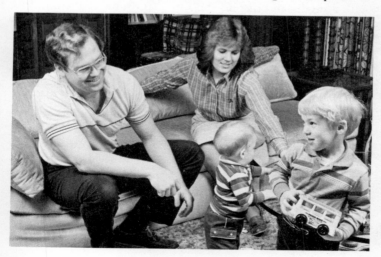

sweaters can be pulled up from the waist. The bunched material covers your breast while the baby conceals your bare midriff. With tops that button, nurse by unbuttoning the bottom ones. If you feel a bit insecure, keep a shawl or blanket handy to wrap around you both. For nighttime feedings, two-piece short or long pajamas are neater to handle than cumbersome night-gowns. There are, however, very lovely nursing gowns on the market that allow for easy exposure of the breast through slits in the fabric.

As far as fabrics are concerned, you won't have time to—nor want to—do any unnecessary ironing. Printed, colorful tops will minimize any leakage and staining, plus your baby will be fascinated by the interesting designs. You may want to think twice about purchasing clothes made of slippery silky materials; you may have a difficult time keeping your baby from sliding away from you!

Adapting Clothes. What about all your one-piece dresses and other nonnursing clothing? Must they be relegated to the back of your closet while you are breastfeeding? If you are handy with a needle and thread, you can adapt some of them to suit your nursing needs. Full slips can have the adjustment clips removed and replaced with an easy-to-open material fastener. For dresses, make a 6″ to 8″ opening along the bust darts or open the seam that runs from the side to the center of your bust. Face each side with tape to prevent fraying; then add hooks or material fasteners. Experiment with both types until you discover which works best for you.

5
Substances That May Affect You and Your Baby

All that you ingest, including alcohol, cigarette smoke, and drugs, passes in some form into your breast milk. When taken in *moderate* amounts, most of these substances pose no danger to you or your nursing baby. But there are exceptions to every rule. To be safe, keep in mind that "binges and babies" don't mix. Excesses of any kind may have a less than desirable effect on your baby and your breastfeeding ability, which is something you don't want.

Caffeine

Ever feel like you are falling apart when you miss your morning cup of coffee? Your body is missing the effect of *caffeine*, a mild stimulant that gives your system that little extra "push" it needs to get going. Caffeine is nonaddictive but by suddenly eliminating it from your diet, headaches, nervousness, and irritability may result. An effective dose of caffeine, one that produces the desired "uplifting" reaction, is considered to be at least 200 milligrams or two cups of strong coffee.

But coffee isn't the only source of caffeine. Teas, too, contain a fair amount—some even more than coffee. Cola drinks are another major source of the substance, with the exception of ginger ales and fruit-flavored beverages. While hot chocolate contains considerably less caffeine, it does have a significant amount of *theobromine* which produces a similar effect. Caffeine can also be found in headache, cold, allergy, and "stay awake" pills as well as certain prescription drugs.

Caffeine and Nursing. What effect can caffeine have on your breastfeeding baby? If you take caffeine in very excessive amounts, your baby may show signs of being jittery or extremely restless. This is rather unlikely to happen, but you could reduce your caffeine intake anyway as a precaution. First, avoid over-consumption; even that "little extra" to heat up your cup begins to add up. Gradually switch to decaffeinated coffee and herb teas; most name-brand soft drinks now sport a caffeine-free double as well. Something you may not have considered is your preparation method. Brewed coffee contains a higher level of caffeine than instant brands, so store away your percolator for a few weeks and see what happens.

Caffeine Levels		
Product	**Portion**	**Amount of Caffeine**
Coffee		
Percolated (roast and ground)	8 oz (1 cup)	75–155 mg
Drip	8 oz	125–155 mg
Instant	8 oz	66 mg
Decaffeinated	8 oz	2–5 mg
Tea		
Black teas	8 oz	28–44 mg
Instant	8 oz	24–131 mg
Soft drinks		
Colas	12 oz	32–65 mg
Pepper drinks	12 oz	32–65 mg
Chocolate		
Hot cocoa	8 oz	5 mg
Milk	1 oz	6 mg
Sweet or dark	1 oz	20 mg
Baking	1 oz	35 mg
Nonprescription drugs		
Analgesic/pain relievers		
Anacin Analgesic, Anacin Maximum Strength, and Anacin-3		32 mg
Cope		32 mg
Excedrin		64.8 mg
Vanquish		33 mg

Caffeine Levels (Cont'd)		
Product	**Portion**	**Amount of Caffeine**
Nonprescription drugs (Cont'd)		
Cold/allergy relief remedies		
Cenegisic		15 mg
Coryban-D		30 mg
Dristan Decongestant and Dristan A–F Decongestant Tablets		16.2 mg
Neo-Synephrine Compounds		15 mg
Sinapils		32.4 mg
Triaminicin		30 mg
Alertness Pills		
No-Doz		100 mg
Vivarin		200 mg
Prescription medicines		
Cafergot and Migralam capsules (migraines)		100 mg
Migral tablets (headaches)		50 mg
Fiorinal (headaches)		40 mg
Espic and Apectol tablets (sedative/ analgesic)		40 mg
Soma Compound (pain reliever and muscle relaxant)		32 mg
Darvon (pain reliever)		32.4 mg

Alcohol

An occasional beer, glass of wine, or cocktail has not been shown to have any ill effects on a nursing baby. In fact a drink while nursing can ease the tensions of the day and enable your milk to let-down more freely. The midevening feeding is a good one because this is when you need relaxation the most, plus the baby will receive less alcohol because the midevening feeding is not as heavy as others. One way to reduce the absorption of alcohol into your bloodstream is to sip your drinks; this gives your liver more time to process it.

When Drinking Becomes Excessive. Alcohol is such a common thing that we rarely consider what it really is—a drug.

Contrary to what you may think, alcohol is a depressant, not a stimulant. It slows down your physical and mental abilities and may even produce unconsciousness when imbibed in sufficient quantities. The amount of alcohol it takes to become drunk varies from person to person according to body weight, amount of food eaten while drinking, and experience with alcohol.

Effects on You and Your Baby. If drinking alcohol becomes a substitute for eating the foods you and your baby need to continue breastfeeding, problems may arise. Your baby may not be getting the necessary nourishment and may become sick from the alcohol that has passed into your milk supply. When you drink heavily, you're hurting yourself as well. Your liver must use up your body's store of vitamins to process the alcohol, and other vitamins will simply pass out of your body due to increased urination. The exact extent to which excessive alcohol consumption can harm your nursing baby is somewhat unclear, but we do know its effects on an unborn baby. *Fetal alcohol syndrome* produces babies with mental, physical, and behavioral abnormalities including hearing defects, hyperactivity, and mental retardation.

Another note—take the time to read the labels of cold remedies and cough syrups. Many contain a good percentage of alcohol as part of the ingredients. We'll talk more about drugs and breastfeeding later on in this chapter.

Effects of Alcohol*		
Quantity	Level in Bloodstream	Reaction
Two shots whiskey (1 oz each) or two 12 oz beers	0.05	Calm
Four shots or beers	0.10	Coordination diminishing
Six shots or beers	0.15	Intoxication
10 shots	0.30	Unconsciousness
20 shots	0.50	Possible death

*Effect on person weighing approximately 150 pounds who is a social drinker.

Cigarette Smoke

Although limited amounts of alcohol won't harm your nursing baby, several of the chemicals—tar, carbon monoxide, and nicotine—in cigarette smoke are known to have ill effects. If you smoke, there's a good chance that amounts of these substances will be found in your breast milk. Nicotine, a common stimulant and probably the major attraction in smoking, is the main culprit. Nicotine suppresses your appetite, making it uncertain whether or not you are eating enough good foods to maintain your milk supply. It may have a similar effect on your baby. Nicotine also causes an increase in heart rate, while carbon monoxide in cigarettes reduces the amount of oxygen able to enter the bloodstream.

"Passive" Smoke Really Isn't Passive. While you may not smoke, your husband or someone else in your family may. Children raised in homes where one or both parents smoke have a higher incidence of upper respiratory infections. Breathing in smoke may increase your baby's heartbeat and blood pressure, putting unnecessary strains on the infant's immature systems.

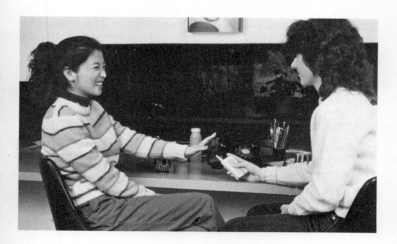

Clearing the Air. If you and your husband have been attempting to stop smoking, this is the time to make a final stand. Quit for your baby's health if not for your own. Make a game of it: The first one caught sneaking a puff has to change baby's diapers for a week. However, if you find that quitting cold turkey makes you so tense and excitable that your milk production lessens or ceases, at least try to cut down or switch to low-tar cigarettes. You may require such a transitional period before being able to stop smoking entirely.

When in public places, such as restaurants, buses, or planes, make arrangements to sit in the nonsmoking section. More and more places are acknowledging the right of nonsmokers to protect their health. Should someone light up while you are with your baby, ask if the person would mind not smoking. Most people will readily comply when a child is involved.

Drugs

If possible, try to avoid all drugs and medications while breastfeeding. While an occasional dose of most medicine shouldn't cause any problems, even aspirin will appear in some level in your breast milk. Naturally if you must take drugs for prolonged or regular periods, the amount in the milk gradually builds up.

With drugs, the main problem is: When does the level of a drug in your milk become so high that it endangers your baby? What might be a minute amount to you could prove to be a substantial dose for your baby. The concentration in which a drug finally appears in your bloodstream and eventually your milk is determined by several factors. The amount of the drug taken is one consideration, but the form also plays a part. A time-release capsule will deliver smaller amounts into your bloodstream at one time, but its effects will be present over a more extended period. Eating also influences the amount. Medicine taken on an empty stomach will pass more quickly into your system. Finally, there's the solubility of the drug—what it dissolves in. Your breast milk is an emulsion of fats and water. If a drug is fat-soluble, it will be more readily incorporated into your milk.

Over-the-Counter and Prescription Drugs

There are more than half a million over-the-counter drugs available to today's consumer. Add to that figure the number of doctor-prescribed-only medications and the numbers become mind-boggling. As mentioned, you should avoid taking either type while breastfeeding, but this may be an impossibility. With over-the-counter drugs, read directions carefully and don't abuse them. If in doubt about their safe use, consult your doctor. As for prescription drugs, make sure the doctor who prescribes them knows that you are breastfeeding. Drug companies are supposed to inform doctors as to whether or not their products can be safely used by lactating women. Ask if there is some way to circumvent your problem 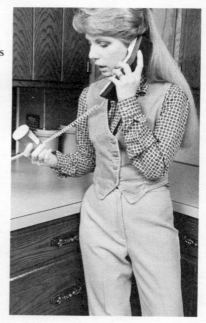 without resorting to medications. Upon discovering that you must take a potentially harmful drug, however, the decision of whether to continue or forego nursing will depend on the importance of the drug to your health. If you are ill, your child will suffer the effects, too. However, if the drug's use will be only short-term, you could express and discard your milk, which will enable you to resume breastfeeding once you're better.

Commonly Abused Drugs		
Drug	**General Effects**	**Method of Taking**
Barbiturates	Depressants; impair normal functioning; addictive; commonly known as sleeping pills	
Barbital		oral
Secobarbital		oral
Pentobarbital		ingestion
Phenobarbital		oral
Amobarbital		oral
Thiopental		ingestion
Narcotics	Sedation and relief of pain; highly addictive and dangerous in some forms	
Morphine		injection
Codeine		oral
Heroin		injection
Meperidine		oral
Stimulants	Feeling of euphoria; increased restlessness; rise in heart rate and blood pressure; artificial highs	
Amphetamine		oral
Methamphetamine		ingestion
Epinephrine		oral
Mescaline		ingestion

Hard Drugs

If over-the-counter drugs are potentially harmful, then taking hard drugs such as cocaine and marijuana is a step toward potential disaster. Most of these drugs affect your mental processes and are habit-forming. In many cases it's not crystal clear exactly how these drugs affect a nursing baby, as most women who use them will not readily admit it. But from the few facts that are documented, it's obvious that hard drugs are something to stay away from—period!

Contraceptives

Nursing mothers have used some oral contraceptives without interfering with their milk supply, but it is still wise to consult your obstetrician for views on the subject. In some women, the Pill has been known to change the nutrient value of breast milk. At times, it may even inhibit lactation. The same hormone used to dry up milk, estrogen, is one of the main components in the Pill. Breastfeeding may supply a little natural contraception of its own; but in addition consider using some barrier method such as diaphragms, spermicidal creams or jellies, or condoms.

6
Breastfeeding While Working

If you are planning to return to work or to find a job soon after your baby's birth, "breast is still best." Breastfeeding assures you of precious moments to spend alone with your baby, moments you may somewhat take for granted while you are home full-time. Working mothers who are convinced of the importance of breastfeeding put a special effort into preserving the closeness of the nursing relationship. You must concentrate on the quality of the time your entire family spends together, because you won't have the quantity any longer.

You'll discover that working even though you're a breastfeeding mother can be relatively easy, but it will take a considerable amount more organization on your part. You can't afford to be late for either. An understanding husband and employer can make the transition period much less tension-provoking and easier on you and your breastfed baby. Learn more about the working mother in *The Evenflo Guide to Working and Caring for Your Baby.*

Why Women Are Returning to Work. Deciding to become a working mother may be one of the most serious decisions you will ever make. While you love your family, you may need a career just as much. Why are mothers working? To utilize their educations, to keep from falling behind in their fields, to relieve feelings of frustration and isolation—these are all common, valid reasons. On the flip side of the coin, other mothers must work because of financial pressures. But whatever your reason for working may be, don't fear that you are alone. Today's mother is the working mother. In 1975, approximately 34% of mothers with children under three years old were in the work force. That figure leapt to 46% in 1983 and has been continuing on the upswing.

As a working mother, you should feel proud about your decision, especially that of continuing to breastfeed. You are trying to do what's best for your baby while at the same time bettering yourself. Rather than the separation being bad for your baby, it may actually be better for both of you. Not being at home 24-hours-a-day may eliminate many tensions and anxieties. You're less apt to be frustrated or annoyed with your baby and may be more appreciative of the time you can spend together. Having a baby shouldn't require sacrifices beyond the call of duty. If you're happier as a working mother, your baby will sense that and be happier, too.

Can It Work? How can I continue to breastfeed when I'm away from home eight hours out of the day? It's really not as impossible as it seems. If your company has in-house day-care

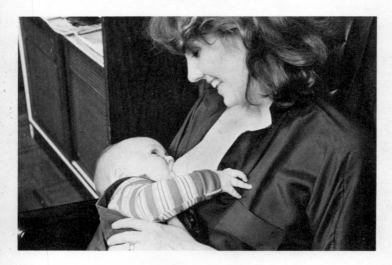

facilities or will allow you to keep your baby in your office, your problems are virtually solved. Unfortunately, such fair-minded companies are few and far between. You could choose part-time or take-home work while your baby is still breastfeeding, but it may not provide the satisfaction and creative stimulation you need. What's the alternative? Work full time and express (manually remove) breast milk for your baby's missed feedings. Expressing milk serves to keep up your supply and relieves the discomfort of engorgement, while ensuring that your baby continues to receive all the benefits of breast milk. It will also maintain the quality of your milk. When your milk remains in your breasts for an extended period, some of the nutrients are reabsorbed. Expressing prevents this from happening by stimulating your breasts to continually produce fresh milk.

You will still have the joys of nursing your baby the last thing before you leave for work and the first thing when you come home, as well as later in the evening and at night. The first week or two may seem hectic, but don't give up. Your family's support and your commitment to breastfeeding will see you through.

Expressing Breast Milk

As you begin working again, you will have to express breast milk by hand or with a pump for the next day's feedings. When you express your milk, you are quickly manually removing it—not allowing your baby to take it at a natural pace. As mentioned, milk can be expressed with your hands or with a pump. You might want to try both methods to determine which suits you best.

Start doing this before you actually return so you'll have a few day's advance supply of milk in your freezer. This will relieve some of the initial pressures you'll face. You will have enough to do trying to reorganize your schedule, plus the tensions resulting from your return may slow your let-down reflex for the first few days, making even the feedings you are nursing somewhat difficult. Just remember to allow yourself extra sleep, and get up a few minutes ahead of time to cope with any unforeseen crises.

Hand Expression

Hand expression may be used to relieve engorgement as well as provide for the missed feedings, though you may find a breast pump more efficient. You should express at least two times during the day: once before leaving for work and again around lunchtime. Don't be concerned if your milk doesn't really flow the first few times; expression takes a little practice to master, plus your milk supply may still be becoming established.

Getting Your Milk to Flow. Before expressing, you will need to stimulate your let-down reflex. Try thinking about your baby or make a tape recording of baby's cry that you can take with you to work. If these fail, warm compresses or massage may do the trick.

Begin by washing your hands thoroughly before handling your breasts. The first thing you'll want to do is work your milk up into the pools beneath your areola. Place your palms flat on your chest with your fingers resting downward on one breast, and press several times on the back portion to move the milk forward. Now rotate your hands so that your fingers are at the base of your breast and push inward toward your nipple about 10 times.

Now you are actually ready to remove your milk. Have a cup or other sterile container handy to catch your breast milk once the flow begins. Place your thumb and forefinger at the base of your areola. As you gently squeeze them together, push backward onto your chest wall. Don't squeeze your nipples or pull at them. Your milk will probably come out in drops at first, then as a fine spray. Rotate your fingers around your areola until all the milk pools in one breast have been emptied; then repeat the procedure on the other side.

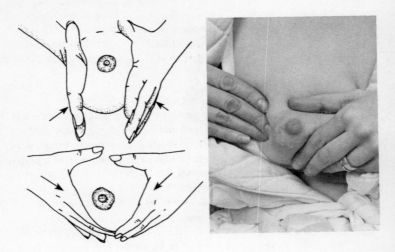

Breast Pumps

During the times you must express milk while at work, you may find a breast pump more convenient to use; it's quicker and the milk flows right into a bottle for easy storage. Two basic pump styles are available. The squeeze bulb-type has been standard, but the newer, syringe-type suction pump may allow for easier, more comfortable expression.

Bulb-type Pumps. To use the bulb-type pump, first apply warm compresses to your breasts; then hand express a few drops of milk to avoid nipple soreness. Wash the pump thoroughly, either by hand or in the dishwasher, before using. Moisten the inside lip of the suction bulb and slide it into place on the narrow end of the horn. Insert the washer in the base of the horn; then screw on the bottle. Squeeze the bulb several times to expel any air that may be inside. To achieve good suction, moisten your breast and the inside edge of the horn before applying the pump. Now squeeze the bulb halfway in and place the broad end of the horn against your breast slightly off center of the nipple so that one side of the horn presses gently near the nipple.

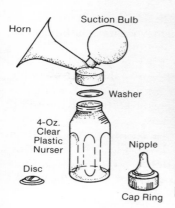

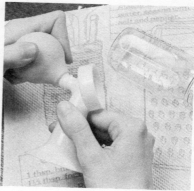

To start the flow, apply some pressure on your breast while gently releasing the bulb. Once the flow has started, relax. Maintain pressure on the bulb until you notice a slowing in your milk flow. To resume the flow, squeeze the bulb gently and at regular intervals. Squeezing too fast may cause nipple irritation. When done, unscrew the bottle from the horn and screw on the cap and disc.

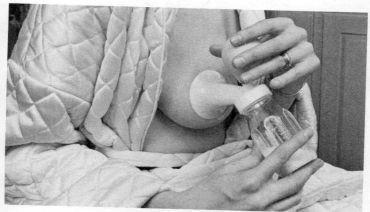

After each use, wash the bulb and horn thoroughly in warm, soapy water; then rinse. You may separate the bulb, horn, and washer for more thorough cleansing.

Syringe-type Pumps. Again, wash all parts of the pump before using. Insert a washer into the cap of the pump assembly. Moistening the washer will allow for a better seal, while prolonging the life of the washer. Screw the bottle onto the pump; then moisten the horn and your breast as previously described. Before placing the horn to your breast, be sure that the handle on the pump is pushed all the way down. Place the horn of the syringe pump against the breast slightly off center of your nipple, so that one side of the horn presses gently near the nipple.

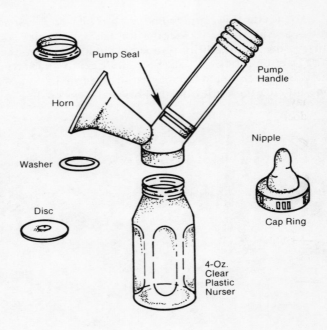

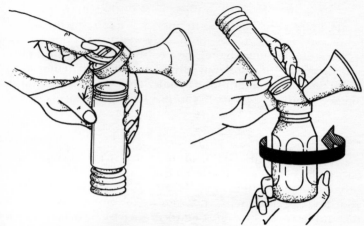

To start the flow, pull up on the pump handle. Do not pull up so hard that you remove the handle from the pump, as this will break the suction. Move the handle up and down as needed to keep the milk flowing, but remember that hard, rapid pumping may prove irritating. If nipple tenderness persists, consult your doctor.

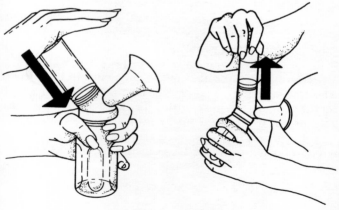

When pumping is complete, remove the pump from the bottle. Place a disc on the bottle and screw a cap ring on tightly for storage. Follow this by thoroughly washing the pump.

Should the pump handle be too difficult to pull out, apply a small amount of petroleum jelly or any edible oil to the pump seal at the bottom of the pump handle. The pump seal should be replaced with a new one if you feel that the pump is losing suction.

Using Expressed Breast Milk

Store your expressed breast milk in a sterile, airtight container; glass and plastic bottles and disposable nurser bags are all suitable for this purpose. Your breast milk can be safely stored in your home or office refrigerator for up to 48 hours. Remember that unlike cow's milk, breast milk is not pasteurized and spoils more rapidly.

If you do not plan to use the fresh breast milk within two days, move the bottle to the freezer. (**Caution:** Never add fresh milk to milk that has already been frozen. This could cause the frozen milk to spoil.) Always mark frozen bottles of milk. Write the date and expression time on a piece of freezer tape. Frozen milk should be used within two weeks. If you can avoid it, don't freeze milk in too large quantities; bottles are easier to handle and result in less waste. Frozen milk may separate, but this presents no nutritional problem. Just be sure to shake up the milk to redistribute the cream before using.

Defrosting Breast Milk. When refrigerated milk is needed for a feeding, hold the container under warm tap water or slowly warm the milk on the stove until it reaches body temperature. Take care not to overheat breast milk, because boiling will destroy the protein. By the same token, never let a bottle warm slowly at room temperature. This practice encourages bacterial growth.

To defrost frozen breast milk, place the container under cool running water and slowly increase the temperature until the frozen milk pulls away from the sides. Then place the container in a pan of water to be warmed. Frozen milk may also be defrosted by placing it in the refrigerator for 24 hours. Once thawed, breast milk should not be refrozen but can be kept refrigerated for two days.

Giving Expressed Milk in a Bottle

You or your husband should acquaint your baby with the idea of milk in a bottle before turning the task over to someone else. Select a glass, plastic, or disposable nurser—there are many varieties from which to choose. The nipple should give milk slowly enough to satisfy your baby's needs, without causing gas and fussiness. The nipple must also adjust to your baby's mouth shape; orthodontic nipples, which simulate the shape of your own nipples, are available to fit most any bottle. For complete information on selecting bottles and nipples, see *The Evenflo Guide to Preparing to Bring Baby Home*.

Feeding. Although you didn't have to bother when breastfeeding, you should test the temperature of the warmed, expressed milk on the inside of your wrist before giving it to your baby. The milk should feel just warm, not hot. Hold your baby in the crook of your arm in a half-sitting, half-lying position. This cuddling is necessary to continue the warmth and security your baby experienced while breastfeeding. Just propping a bottle in your baby's mouth does not provide the love and care needed.

Hold the bottle so that the breast milk always covers the nipple. This prevents your baby from sucking in air that can cause an upset stomach. It's not unlikely that your baby may refuse the bottle the first few times it's offered because it just doesn't seem "right." This is where lots of patient coaxing will have to come into play. The flow of the bubbles will let you know when your infant begins feeding. Slow-rising bubbles may indicate that your baby is having difficulty, so loosen the screw ring to ease the flow.

Stop feeding as soon as the baby loses interest, the same as when breastfeeding. Don't try to force-feed the entire bottle. If any milk is left, discard it.

Supplemental Bottles

Once your lactation is firmly established, about three to four weeks after birth, your baby may occasionally skip a feeding of breast milk. Once you launch full-force into your work responsibilities, you may find it difficult to pump all you need each day. In this case it may be best for you to use expression to relieve discomfort; then supplement with formula for the missed feedings. While formula may not be as good as breast milk, it may be a more realistic alternative than suffering with a disjointed work schedule or trying to pacify a hungry baby.

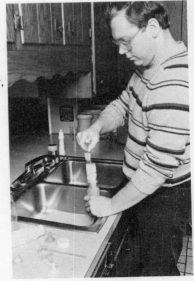

Formulas are available in liquid concentrate, powder, and ready-to-use varieties. Your doctor will be able to recommend one suitable for your baby's needs. Since formula will only be used for one or two feedings, preparing it by the single bottle method may be most practical. Wash your hands with soap and water; then thoroughly wash the bottle, nipple, and accessories in hot, soapy water or in

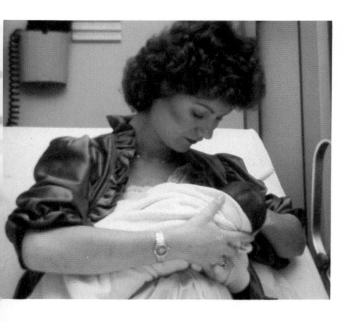

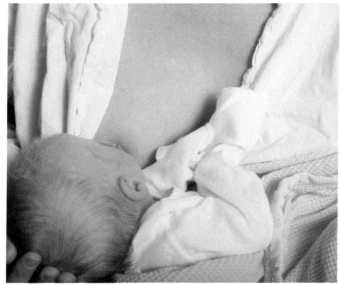

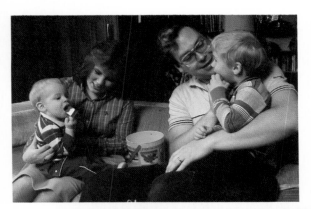

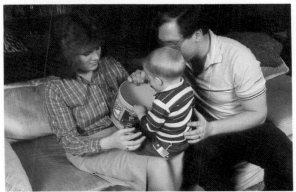

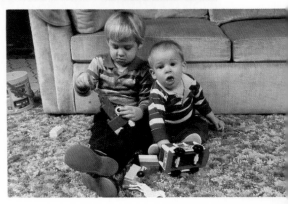

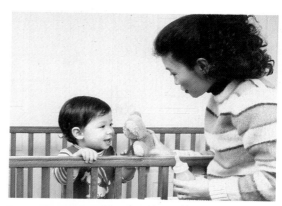

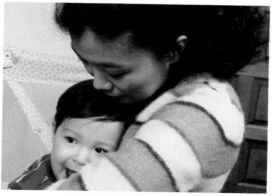

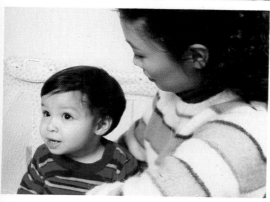

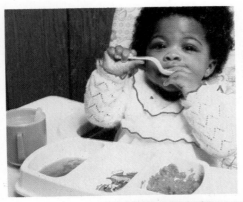

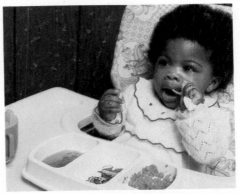

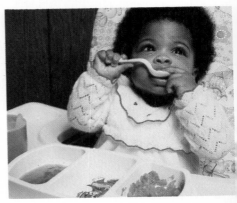

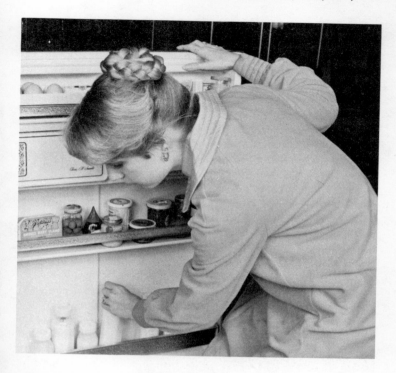

the dishwasher. Squeeze the water through the nipple hole to make sure it's open. Prepare the formula as directed by the manufacturer, washing the top of the can before opening. Screw on the nipple, nipple disc, and screw ring. Store the bottles in the refrigerator. Warm the bottle by using an electric bottle warmer or just place the bottle in warm water.

Who Will Care for My Baby?

If you are working full time, finding someone to care for your baby in your absence is an ultimate necessity. It's a decision you and your husband should make very carefully, for your baby's sake. Besides requiring love and security, babies also need continuity of care. They must have one person with whom they can develop strong bonds. This means the fewer changes in the person caring for your baby, the better. But what type of care should my baby get? Unfortunately there is no perfect child care arrangement. Each has its pros and cons. It's your job to evaluate all options, comparing convenience and quality with cost. To narrow down the field, begin by making a choice between the two main types of care—individual and group.

Individual Care

Your husband is a natural for the job of taking care of the baby. More and more fathers are taking advantage of paternity leaves or are using vacation time to be home with their babies. Some find that they enjoy taking care of the baby so much that they become full-time househusbands. Of course, this arrangement isn't for every family, especially where economic factors prevail. Your husband could also switch to working a shift opposite to yours, but this often results in marital tensions.

Mothers, grandparents, and in-laws are also baby-care favorites. Relatives are often more flexible in their schedules and are likely to share your ideals and values. In most cases, they're also easier on your budget; professional child care can become expensive. If a relative does offer to baby-sit, it's an option you should definitely consider.

Baby-sitters. Housekeepers and baby nurses are two other alternatives, but the most popular type of individualized care is undoubtedly the baby-sitter. When choosing a sitter, you and your husband must be on the lookout for someone who understands a baby's needs. Maturity should probably be at the top of your list of qualifications. There are some extremely mature 18-year-olds and a few very childish 40-year-olds, so don't evaluate on the basis of age alone. Look for reliability, patience, cheerfulness, and love of children. While not a necessity, a baby-sitter with a car can be a blessing should an emergency arise.

Advertisements, employment agencies, and the recommendations of friends are all useful ways of locating a suitable sitter. Don't decide on the basis of a phone conversation alone; call each likely possibility in for a personal interview.

Working with Your Sitter. Once you choose a sitter, give the person time to become acquainted with your baby. Plan a few nights out with your husband as "trial runs." One rule of thumb: Don't sneak out on a sleeping baby. While you save yourself from ear-piercing cries, your baby may come to associate sleep with your disappearance and may develop irregular sleeping habits. No matter how old the baby is, always say "good-bye" and that you'll return. Your baby will eventually latch onto the idea that you will come back. Baby may cling to you and cry as you go out the door, but the "flood" should only last for a short while.

Inform the sitter that you are breastfeeding, and give details on how to defrost and feed expressed milk. Make sure you leave your work telephone numbers as well as those of your doctor, the fire department, and the police. Point out important features of your house and the location of fire extinguishers and first aid kits. Be sure to supply your sitter with one other important piece of information—when you'll be returning.

Group Care

Group care may take the form of family day-care or the more common day-care centers. Family day-care usually centers around a woman—usually a mother herself—who takes care of children in her home. Only in certain states, for example Wyoming and Washington, are these state-regulated, so you must do considerable checking. Visit the home, find out who the other children are, and discuss what the care includes. While the quality may vary, family day-care may be the only alternative economically feasible for your family.

Day-care Centers. You may have to shop around a little before you find a day-care program that accepts infants; many only take children who are already toilet trained. Day-care

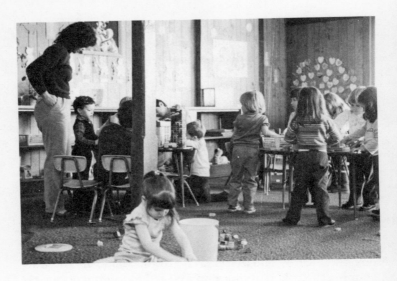

centers have the advantages of providing continuity of care, a fair degree of professionalism, intensive social interaction, and better regulation. Make sure the one you select is licensed by the appropriate governmental agency in your community to ensure at least minimal standards. A good center not only cares for children, but helps them learn and grow mentally as well as physically.

To provide for adequate attention, the program should have two qualified staff members for every four to six babies and toddlers. In addition, the program should provide clean and safe facilities, appropriate play materials, and nourishing meals. Remember that since you are breastfeeding, you'll have to provide the center with a supply of your milk. You may feel uneasy at first about leaving your baby with complete strangers in a strange environment, but the staff should be willing to discuss your reservations with you and plan how the center can best benefit your baby. If the center is unwilling to involve parents, look elsewhere.

Checklist for Judging a Day-care Center

- Does the person caring for the children really care about your child as an individual?
- Does the care giver treat each child as his or her own, talking to each child while bathing or changing diapers, holding each child when feeding, or "teaching," and paying attention to each child's temperament and development?
- Is the home or center safe and healthful with room for children's play and care, fresh air, reasonable cleanliness, and free of safety and accident hazards?
- Are your suggestions for the care of your baby welcomed and listened to?
- Do the care givers and children seem to be happy, alert, and enjoying themselves?
- Are children of various ages segregated (i.e., infants, toddlers, older children)?
- Are you welcome to visit at any time, with or without telling in advance that you are coming?
- Has the care giver had a medical examination to show that he or she has no disease that your baby could contract and is strong and healthy enough to care for children?
- Is there a telephone which the care giver can use to reach you or to call for help in an emergency?
- In the event of an emergency, are there staff members trained in CPR or first aid who can provide immediate care?
- What is the policy of the center on caring for sick children? Are sick children segregated from well ones?
- Is there a sufficient staff available at all times during the day?
- Does the center provide consistency in physical surroundings and personnel—regularity of meals and naptimes, arrangement of furniture, and hours of staff?
- Are the children taught controls, what is permissible and what is not, and praised for correct behavior?

Managing Your Life

Trying to juggle breastfeeding, work, and household duties may send you reeling. The days just aren't long enough and the stacks of things that need to be done keep increasing. What can you do? Basically, you have to realize that you can't do everything—it's humanly impossible, even for a "supermom." Establish priorities and get help—from your husband, the babysitter, and friends. Chores can wait; your baby can't.

Make a list of the things that need to be done, according to their priority. Delegate what you can to others, and just concentrate on the essential tasks—particularly those involving the baby. Don't forget to leave blocks of free time just for yourself. You still need to sleep and eat, even if you can't see how it fits into your schedule! If you're tired and undernourished, you'll have difficulty nursing or expressing milk for your baby, not to mention that it will affect your efficiency at work. So take the advice we've reiterated time and time again, and take care of yourself.

7
When Problems Arise

You and your husband naturally want to do what's best for your baby. Your decision to breastfeed your baby is a good example of your care and concern. More than likely, your choice was at least partially influenced by the health benefits breastfeeding offers for both you and your baby. Nevertheless, these benefits, plus other precautions you may take, cannot prevent some feeding problems from arising. Your baby may develop an upset tummy, or your breasts may become swollen or irritated. Fortunately, these problems are not serious. Everyone experiences at least some of them during baby's first year. However, you have the extra incentive of your breastfeeding commitment to help see you through.

Crying

Let's face it—babies cry! It is their best and most frequently used form of communication; one to which you as parents eventually become accustomed. You learn that not all of your infant's cries indicate hunger. Sometimes these cries will mean that your infant is hurt, tired, or lonely and misses you. At times such as these don't worry that you are spoiling your child if you respond to the cries. Many studies show that parents' immediate answering to babies' tears has no ill effect on the children. By quickly answering baby's cries you are showing that you love and care for your infant. Baby learns to trust you and comes to know that you are there when needed. As time goes by, your child

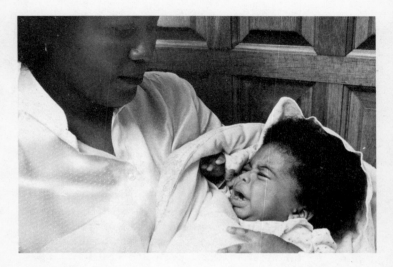

develops new and better ways to communicate these wants; thus, crying takes on new meanings.

Hunger Cries

Occasionally, baby may continue crying after a feeding session. The cries could be telling you that baby is still hungry and wants to suckle a little longer. If this is the case, try extending your nursing periods. Feeding your baby more for a longer length of time usually does the trick.

Is Baby Sick?

If crying is the only symptom, the answer is usually no. However, there are times when you should be concerned. When baby feeds poorly, becomes lethargic, develops a temperature, has diarrhea, vomits, or is simply not acting right, contact your doctor for treatment.

For more on baby illnesses, refer to *The Evenflo Guide to Your Baby's Health from birth to one year.*

Spitting Up

Spitting up, or regurgitation, is a common feeding problem. Some babies always spit up during or after a feeding. Others never regurgitate. Most, however, fall into the middle category of those who occasionally spit up. The milk seems to overflow from the baby's mouth and is often curdled from normal stomach action. This is really not a health problem; it is just messy. So keep a diaper or washcloth handy for quick cleanups.

There are several tricks to reduce the amount of spitting up. Unfortunately none of them is guaranteed to work all of the time, and most babies will continue some spitting up, even when all of the following tricks are used:

- Try to ensure that your baby does not take in too much milk at one time.
- Burp your baby carefully midway through feeding, at the end of feeding, and a few minutes after feeding.
- Prop up your baby's infant seat or cradle a few inches so that your baby's head is tilted forward over the stomach for 10 to 15 minutes after each nursing session.
- Remember that there is no cause for alarm as long as your baby is developing favorably.

Colic

Some babies have attacks of crying nearly every evening, usually between 6:00 and 10:00 *p.m.* During such attacks, babies frown, their faces redden, and they draw up their legs. They scream loudly—a cry quite different from the cries of hunger or loneliness. Crying may continue from 2 to 20 minutes, even when the baby is picked up and comforted. The attack may end suddenly, or soft crying may last a few minutes after the hard crying stops. Just as the baby is about to fall asleep, another attack may occur. Gas may rumble in the stomach and be passed through the rectum.

No one knows what causes such attacks. Many feel that it is an intestinal problem similar to gas pains that you as an adult may experience. Others think it is the result of baby's taking too much air into the stomach. Still others assert that baby's internal system is not yet mature enough; therefore, your infant feels uncomfortable.

Whatever the cause, many of the characteristics of colic are universal. Colic attacks usually come at the same time every day. At other times of the day, the infant is happy, alert, eats well, and gains weight.

What can you do to soothe your baby? During an attack, holding your infant across your knees on the stomach often will give some comfort. There is little you can do except comfort your baby until the attack stops. Be sure the baby isn't just hungry, wet, or lonely, and that no piece of clothing is uncomfortable. Most important, remember that colic does not interfere with

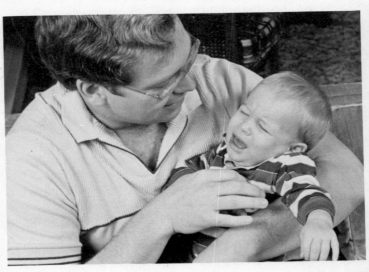

your baby's general health and growth, and that your baby will grow out of it around 12 to 16 weeks of age. Colicky babies do annoy their mothers and fathers and anybody living in the household. Remind everyone that it is not the baby's fault, it is not your fault, and the baby will get over it. If the colic becomes a real problem, it is worth a special trip or call to the doctor, who may be able to prescribe a medicine to make the baby rest more comfortably.

Bowel Movements

Your baby's first bowel movements are sticky and greenish black. This substance, called meconium, is a combination of dead cells from the liver, pancreas, and gall bladder. The meconium, which was formed in the intestines, must be eliminated before normal bowel movements can occur. Fortunately, your colostrum helps the process along.

After a week or two the bowel movements will become looser and lighter. In fact, the stools of your breastfed baby will differ from those of the bottlefed baby. So don't worry that your baby has diarrhea. Those yellow, soft, and seedy stools are not at all unusual.

The frequency of your baby's bowel movements will also differ. Your baby may have anywhere from one movement every three or four days to five or six movements a day. Also don't be surprised if your baby grunts and pushes during a bowel movement. Breastfed babies naturally act this way. It is not a sign of constipation.

If your baby's bowel movements seem looser than usual, look to your own diet for a possible cause. Just as the taste of what you eat, like garlic, can be tasted by baby, so too can the foods you eat, like cabbage, affect bowel movements. So to eliminate these looser stools, adjust your own diet by removing the offending foods.

Vaginal Bleeding

During the first few weeks after birth you may notice a small amount of vaginal bleeding when you are changing your daughter's diapers. This is quite common, so there is little need for concern. While your daughter was still in your womb some of your hormones passed through your placenta into her system. This "false menstruation" is her system's way of adjusting.

Diarrhea

Your baby has a mild form of diarrhea if bowel movements are more frequent, looser, or green in color. Usually treatment is simple, quick, and effective as long as you contact your baby's doctor for immediate treatment. A change in your diet most probably will solve the problem.

Severe diarrhea in children under the age of one is usually due to bacteria or a virus in their systems. It is very important for you to contact your baby's physician at the first signs of a watery bowel movement. Your baby needs to regain all the fluids lost. In many cases, it may be necessary to discontinue any formula feeding and give only clear fluids or breast milk until the diarrhea clears up.

Constipation

Constipation exists when your infant's bowel movements are hard, dry, and difficult to pass, no matter how frequent or infrequent they may be. Breastfed babies seldom experience constipation, but when they do, changes in your diet will eliminate any discomfort your baby feels. Do not use mineral oil, castor oil, adult laxatives, or enemas without medical advice.

Blood in Bowel Movements

Slight blood streaking on the outside of a bowel movement is usually caused by a small sore or fissure in your baby's anus and is not a cause for alarm. You can often cure the fissure and the bleeding by keeping your infant's stools soft by adjusting your diet. If bleeding or hard bowel movements persist, your doctor will be able to help. Do not delay medical attention if there is bloody diarrhea or if fresh blood or clots are passed with the bowel movements.

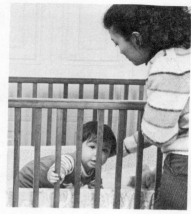

Diaper Rash

Bowel movements are irritating to your baby's skin, especially when they stay in contact with the skin for a long time. You can prevent irritating diaper rash by changing your baby's diapers frequently. Also rinse baby's bottom with clean water at each diaper change or use baby wipes. If you use cloth diapers, it is important that you rinse the cloth diapers thoroughly after each

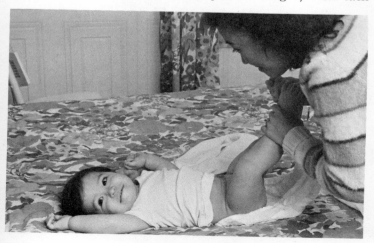

washing. This eliminates any lingering detergent or bleach residues. Finally, try applying a protective layer of ointment (like zinc oxide paste) to any irritated area.

If your baby gets a diaper rash in spite of these precautionary measures, you should try the following suggestions. Leave off plastic pants or plastic-covered disposable diapers, except when absolutely necessary. Using two or more cloth diapers at naptime and at night will make this less messy. Completely uncover your baby's diaper area for a few hours each day (naptime or early evening is most convenient). Put a few diapers under baby to prevent soiling. Finally, apply a thin layer of a protective ointment to any irritated area after cleansing at each diaper change.

Occasionally diaper rash will cause baby more discomfort than usual. You can soak such a rash with a washcloth or towel wrung out in warm water. Remember to keep the rash clean by washing it with mild soap and water twice a day. If it doesn't improve in a day or two, contact your baby's doctor.

Mother's Problems

Despite all of the exercises done prenatally to toughen your nipples and prepare your breasts for nursing, you may still feel some discomfort. Your breasts might become slightly sensitive to the touch or your nipples might begin to crack. Whatever your complaint, try not to become upset. Neither you nor your baby will benefit from any undue disturbance to your nursing routine. Remember that you are in good company. Most, if not all, nursing mothers experience some type of minor soreness when they begin to nurse. Others even develop small problems well into breastfeeding. Fortunately, your commitment to breastfeeding helps you solve any problems or work around them.

Engorgement (Swollen Breasts)
When there is too much milk in your breasts, they are said to be swollen or engorged. Swollen breasts may occur during the

first three to five days of nursing or when you miss a nursing period. Your doctor or nursing instructor usually mentions swelling of breast tissues, increased blood circulation, and the heaviness of your fresh milk supply as the causes. You know that your breasts are engorged if they appear hard and hurt when you touch them. You should also feel a constricting sensation.

If you allow your baby to regulate feeding and eliminate supplementary bottles for the first 30 days, you can prevent engorgement. This encourages your baby to nurse more intently. Because of the increased suckling time, baby empties your breasts and engorgement is no longer a problem.

Once your breasts do become engorged, you can easily relieve any discomfort by trying one or a combination of some of the following suggestions.

Ask your doctor about your taking aspirin one hour before a nursing session. This tends to alleviate any discomfort you may feel when baby touches your breast.

Try supporting your breast with a firm-support nursing bra, but make certain that it does not bind you. A constricting nursing bra only makes you feel more uncomfortable.

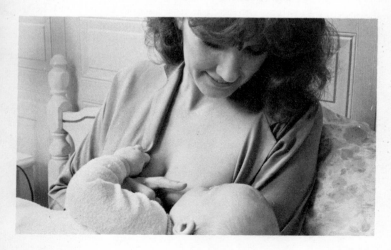

Both extremes of temperature also bring relief. Heat expands the milk ducts, thereby aiding the let-down reflex. Cold relieves the swelling and discomfort of your breasts. Try ice packs, heating pads, a carefully wrapped hot-water bottle, or even a warm towel at intervals. Some women have also found comfort simply by enjoying a warm, relaxing shower.

Expressing your milk by hand or by pump eases any swelling. Just express a small amount before each feeding. This softens your breasts and makes it easier for your baby to nurse. Review the method for expressing milk in Chapter 6. Generally engorgement should fade within 24 to 48 hours.

You might also want to ask your physician about the use of prescription drugs to alleviate any discomfort and swelling. Two choices are stilbestrol, an inhibitor of milk production, and oxytocin, which you already know aids the let-down reflex.

Sore Nipples

We have already lightly touched upon your brief feelings of discomfort during the early days of breastfeeding. By now you know that as soon as your milk comes in, the discomfort usually disappears. For those times when your nipples become cracked, chapped, or overly uncomfortable, a telephone call to your doctor starts you well on the way to correcting this commonplace problem.

One of the first suggestions your doctor most probably should make concerns your baby's grasp of the breast. You'll be asked to check that your baby is sucking on both your nipple and areola. Baby's nursing on only your nipple may be the cause of your soreness. If your infant has not been correctly nursing, review the method for getting baby to feed. (See Chapter 3.)

If you are wearing a nursing bra, remove the plastic linings in the cups. While the plastic is effective in preventing embarrassing leakage, it traps moisture that can cause irritation and chafing. The same holds true if you are using nursing shields or other absorbent pads. Try changing the pads more often.

Do not moisturize or clean your nipples with any products that could irritate or dry them. Avoid substances such as witch hazel, petroleum jelly, soap, and alcohol. If you must moisturize your breasts, use only creams which are mild and fragrance free.

Air dry your nipples when possible. Expose them to the air when you are staying at home. You might also try sleeping with the flaps of your nursing bra open. Finally, ease sore nipples during breastfeeding by using nipple shields.

Plugged Ducts

In Chapter 1, we mentioned that milk ducts can become blocked if your nursing bra is too tight. Unlike some discomforts, plugged or clogged ducts can occur intermittently throughout nursing. When do you know if you have plugged ducts? You usually will be able to find a small lump on your breast that hurts when you or anyone else touches it. These usually occur in the section of your breast closest to your armpit. It is especially important for you to immediately get medical assistance. Your physician can recommend a treatment that will offset any chance of a breast infection or a breast abscess.

Here are some suggestions your doctor may advise you to try. As with many nursing problems, remember that continued breastfeeding helps to alleviate discomfort and eliminate the problem. So follow these suggestions and stay in touch with your physician.

The most important point is to ensure that the affected breast is always emptied at a feeding. Extend your feeding times; let your baby suckle more often and for longer periods of time. You might also try offering the breast with the plugged duct first, keeping in mind that baby empties the breast offered first. If it is not possible to offer the sore breast, express milk from it until the duct unclogs. Expressing your milk maintains milk production and eases any uncomfortable feelings. Some women also use an expression technique of moving the milk from the periphery of the breast toward the nipple in the area that is blocked. One preventative measure is to massage your breasts during and after each nursing session.

To lessen any discomfort you feel when your infant touches your breast, try changing feeding positions. This takes the pressure off of the sore part of your breast.

If your nipples are caked, a careful wash with sterilized water removes any substances discharged from your affected breast.

Breast Infection and Abscess

If a breast infection (mastitis) is going to occur, it usually does so during the first month after baby's birth. You may have a headache, fever, and tender, swollen breasts that are red and hot to the touch. Bacteria is the cause of the infection in most cases.

It is important that mastitis be treated within the first 24 hours. Contact your doctor at the first sign of discomfort and then go straight to bed. Your physician will prescribe a treatment similar to the one for breast engorgement—heat, a firm nursing bra, and your baby's complete emptying of the breast—together with antibiotics to fight the infection.

If a breast infection is not treated immediately, pus gathers in one area and an abscess forms. These can more readily occur in women who are diabetic, and thus more prone to infections. Your doctor will usually prescribe antibiotics, which in most cases are sufficient to clear up the problem.

Breastfeeding during Illness

From the discussion of mother's problems, you now know that in most cases you can still nurse your baby when you're ill. Usually baby has been exposed to your germs before you can see or feel any of the symptoms. However, you should check with both your doctor and your baby's doctor when diarrhea, fever, or vomiting occur.

8
Changing Nutritional Needs

For the first six months of your baby's life, breast milk is the only food that will be required. It provides all the vitamins (with the exception of vitamin D) and nutrients needed for growth and development. How long you continue to breastfeed beyond this time depends on you and your baby. But sooner or later, you'll have to begin thinking about how and when to wean your baby.

Weaning is the process by which your baby stops depending solely on your breast milk for nourishment, marking the first movement away from the intimate nursing relationship you've shared. It's the point where baby's eating habits transform from those of an infant to the more varied and self-regulated ones of a child. The process actually begins to some extent when you start supplementing your baby's feedings with solids. However, complete weaning won't occur until your infant stops breast-feeding entirely. For more information on infant nutrition, refer to *The Evenflo Guide to Your Baby's Health from birth to one year.*

Introducing Solid Foods

More than likely, the first step you'll take toward weaning is to start your baby on solid foods. Don't try to stop nursing altogether and force solids into the baby's diet; it will be too much of a physical strain on your baby.

Opinions among pediatricians vary greatly about exactly when to begin solids. Some believe in starting as early as the fourth month, though most recommend waiting for a full six months. Usually it depends a lot on when your baby indicates that it's time. You may hear some mothers boasting that their babies were eating solids during their first month. They may have been, but that doesn't mean it's a sound practice to follow. Babies initially need the nutrients found in breast milk. Eating solids may deter them from nursing as much as they should and deprive them of the vitamins and minerals they so desperately need at this stage in their lives. Also a baby younger than three months is not physically ready to tackle solids because the digestive system is not that highly developed.

How to Begin

Introduce solids while your baby is still nursing regularly. In fact, nurse before you try to offer the solid. A baby who is not in the middle of hunger pangs will be more receptive to something new. When you start limiting the breastfeedings, feed the solid first so nursing is reduced. Begin gradually, with 1 teaspoon once a day; the early morning feeding is a good one with which to start. If your husband complains about being left out when you breastfeed, here's his chance to help out.

Keep It Simple. Try just one new food at a time and feed it for several days. These should be pure, simple foods. Use pure rice cereal, not mixed cereals, and applesauce, rather than fruit dessert. New foods may cause allergic reactions such as vomiting, skin rash, diarrhea, or constipation in a few infants. By starting only one new food every four or five days and by using simple foods, you can more easily determine which food is at the root of the problem. If your baby does have a reaction, stop the food and then reintroduce it in small amounts a few months later. Continued allergic responses should be reported to your doctor. If your baby seems happy and unaffected, however, you can be fairly sure that you can use that food in the future without any problems.

Foods to Limit. Certain foods are known allergy producers in some infants. These include the
following: cow's milk, egg whites,
wheat, corn, pork, fish and
shellfish, citrus fruits and juices,
and strawberries. Although you
don't have to avoid these
entirely, do watch
for any reaction
when baby eats any
of these foods. While your
baby may look longingly at
nuts, raisins, or popcorn,
don't feed them. Hard bits
may become lodged in your
baby's throat and cause
choking. Honey is also not
recommended for infants. Recent findings
show that honey may contain spores of botulism bacteria and
that these spores may be dangerous to your baby.

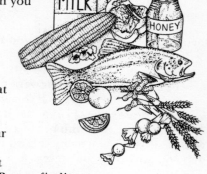

What about candy and other sweets? Candy, cookies, sugar, and soft drinks have little nutritional value. They are also bad for developing teeth and may spoil your baby's appetite for more nutritious foods. Use them only occasionally or eliminate them altogether.

Homemade versus Commercial Baby Food. Should you buy commercially prepared foods for your baby or make your own? Both will provide your baby with good nutrition; therefore, it all depends upon what you prefer. Essentially, baby foods are foods that have been strained to a fine consistency. Should you pay for something you can do yourself with a blender—at little or no cost?

Besides expense, what about the controversy over additives found in baby foods? For years manufacturers were adding sugar and salt to their preparations, not for the baby's palate, but for mom, who was sampling the food! Studies show that the need for salt is an acquired taste, that babies under seven months old can't really differentiate between salted and unsalted foods. As a result, most baby food manufacturers have removed these additives from their products. You may see these advertised as "new, natural baby foods."

Commercial baby foods do have one major point in their favor—they're convenient. All you have to do is open the jar, perhaps warm it, and the food is ready to serve. If you are a working mother with limited free time, these extra few moments may be a great inducement toward the use of such foods.

Starting from Scratch. If you want to make your own baby food, or at least some of it, you'll find that it's really not all that difficult or time-consuming. You can use most of the table foods your family eats, but avoid canned fruits and vegetables which may contain overly high levels of salt. If you must use canned or frozen products, rinse them to wash off some of the salt prior to cooking or heating.

Fruits are an easy food to start with when making your own food. Peel a banana, apple, pear, or peach; slice it finely; mix with juice or milk; and blend. You have instant baby food with no artificial ingredients. You can do the same with meat and vegetables by pureeing them at high speed. Do, however, scoop out baby's portion before seasoning the food for the rest of the family.

Increasing the Feedings. After a month or so, start offering solids between nursings and increase the amount to several tablespoons. Here's a typical schedule you can follow that combines breastfeeding with solids. However, it's not unlikely that your baby's doctor may have a special feeding program; opinions on this matter do vary greatly from physician to physician.

Helping Baby Eat

Don't laugh at the cartoon of the food-splattered mother or father unsuccessfully trying to spoon cereal into a baby's mouth.

| | Daily Solid Food Introduction Schedule | | |
Month	Breastfeedings Daily	Number of Solid Feedings Daily	Amount of Solids Per Feeding
First	6–8	0	
Second	6–8	0	
Third	5–6	0	0–1 tsp
Fourth	5–6	0	1–2 tsps
Fifth	4–5	1–2	1 tsp
Sixth	4–5	4–5	2–3 tbsps
Seventh	4–5	3–4	6–7 tbsps
Eighth	3–4	3–4	6–7 tbsps
Ninth	3–4	3–4	7–10 tbsps
Tenth	3–4	3–4	7–10 tbsps
Eleventh	3–4	3–4	7–10 tbsps
Twelfth	3–4	3–4	7–10 tbsps

Source—U.S. Dept. of Agriculture/Food and Nutrition Service pamphlet, *What Shall I Feed My Baby?*

Tomorrow, it could be you! Your baby may decide that solids are more fun to play with than to eat. If baby is too young to sit in a high chair, hold your infant in a slightly reclined position in the crook of your arm. Wear an apron and put a bib on baby; the first few attempts are bound to be messy.

A small or demitasse spoon will make feeding easier. Special baby spoons are also available, some with rubber bowls that feel good against baby's tender gums. Fill the spoon about half full and touch it to your baby's lips. When the lips part, put the spoon on the center of your baby's tongue, but not so far back as to cause choking. Draw out the spoon, wiping the food on the bottom of baby's upper lip. Even better, just touch the spoon to baby's lips and let baby suck off the food. This will improve lip control. At first your baby may push out the food with the tongue or even spit or blow it out. Eventually, however, your infant will take a little into the mouth and swallow it.

As soon as your little one is able, encourage baby to help you handle the spoon during feedings. Sit behind so that baby

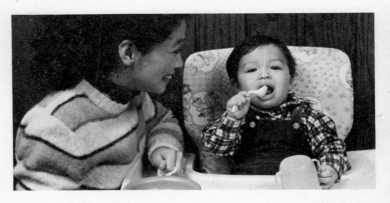

can hold onto the spoon or onto your hand to learn the movements. This may slow you down and cause a bit of slopping, but your baby will be eating without your help sooner.

Whatever you do, don't prod your baby to eat. Even babies can have some definite likes and dislikes. If yours repeatedly rejects a food, substitute something else. Aside from breast milk, no one food is indispensable. Another pointer: When babies seal their mouths, it means they've had enough. Don't try to sneak in that last little spoonful. It can be the start of a vicious cycle of fights when feeding. And if upset, your child will eat less and possibly have trouble keeping it down.

Storing Baby Food

When purchasing prepared baby food, always check the package date and try to use it before the recommended time for the best quality. Feed your baby from a serving dish rather than from a jar, particularly if you think you will have leftovers. Your baby's saliva on the spoon carries germs and will cause the food to become watery. Refrigerate any unused portions.

For homemade foods, try to use them soon after preparation if possible—fruits and vegetables within two to three days and meats within one day. The easiest way to store baby food for any length of time is to freeze it in individual portions. Place 1 to 2 tablespoons of food in each compartment of an ice cube tray and freeze them. Pop out the frozen cubes of food, put it into plastic bags, and store in the freezer. Baby food frozen in this manner will keep for one to two months. To use, place one or more cubes in a cup or a small dish and heat over water. Once thawed, the food cannot be refrozen.

Starter Foods

When starting your baby on solids, cereals are usually the first food. These are followed by fruits, vegetables, and meats as the weeks go by until your baby is eating a balanced diet.

Cereals. Cereals are quite easy to digest, so they're ideal for baby's introduction to solids. Begin, perhaps in baby's fifth month if the doctor so recommends, with an iron-fortified, single grain cereal. Rice is mild and less likely to cause allergic reactions than wheat or corn. For the first feeding, mix the cereal with enough formula, milk, or water to make it look like creamed soup. Start with a spoonful and gradually increase the amount, adding other grain cereals such as oats and barley as you do.

Fruits. Because they are simple to prepare and eat, you'll probably introduce fruits and juices next. Just mash or chop finely, add liquid, and blend. Or you can use commercially prepared fruits. Remember to serve only single fruits first to determine if there will be any allergic reaction.

Vegetables. The first vegetables you feed your baby should be smooth and liquid in consistency. To best preserve nutrients when preparing vegetables yourself, steam, bake, or boil them in a small amount of water until they are just done. Peel and remove seeds if necessary. For a finer consistency, rub the vegetables through a strainer or puree in the blender. Use the juices from cooking as the blending liquid. Most physicians recommend starting with yellow vegetables such as carrots, squash, and sweet potatoes. Add green vegetables later.

Solid Food Progression Schedule

Age in Months	Food Consistency	Grains					Fruits		Vegetables	Dairy	Protein					Finger Foods
		Cereals	Toast	Noodles	Macaroni	Rice	Whole	Juice		Cheese	Eggs	Meat	Poultry	Dried beans	Dried peas	
Three																
Four																
Five	strained	*X														
Six	strained	X					X		X			X		X	X	
Seven	finely chopped	X	X				X		X			X		X	X	
Eight	chopped	X	X				X	X	X	X		X	X	X	X	
Nine	chopped	X	X				X	X	X			X	X	X	X	X
Ten	chopped	X	X	X	X	X	X	X	X	X		X	X	X	X	X
Eleven	chopped / table food	X	X	X	X	X	X	X	X	X		X	X	X	X	X
Twelve	chopped / table food	X	X	X	X	X	X	X	X	X	X	X	X	X	X	X

*If recommended by baby's doctor.

Protein Foods. Meats, dairy products, and beans (legumes) are all good sources of protein for your baby. In addition to protein, iron and other nutrients are supplied by beans and meats. Like vegetables, protein foods should be pureed for the first feedings.

To prepare meats, fish, and poultry, remove all skin and fat; then bake, broil, stew, or braise. Take care to remove any and all bones. Grind or puree the meat in a blender. You may want to start your baby on either veal or lamb because these are less likely to cause an allergic reaction.

Cooked dried beans, peas, and lentils can substitute for meat at some feedings. Prepare them without any seasonings, including butter. If you have a food mill, put the beans through to remove the skins and mash the edible portion.

Cheese, yogurt, and cottage cheese are all protein supplements, but use them cautiously if your baby shows any allergy toward milk. Do not start these foods until baby's physician has suggested adding whole milk to the diet.

Finger Foods. Babies enjoy trying to eat by themselves with their fingers. When you see that your baby is trying to attempt this, give him crackers, bits of bread or toast, cubed cheese, or pieces of banana or peeled apple. Avoid small, dried foods or foods with strings such as celery.

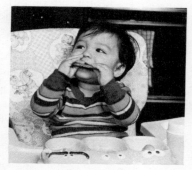

Changes in Bowel Movements

While breastfeeding, your baby's bowel movements were usually slightly loose with no unpleasant odor. Suddenly they may turn pastier or be colored orange, red, or green. These are the effects of the addition of solids to the diet. Monitor your baby's bowel movements somewhat while introducing the new foods in case one should cause a reaction.

How to Wean Your Baby from the Breast

There is no "right" time to stop your baby from breastfeeding. Some mothers nurse for only three or four months, while others continue until their child is two years old. Usually, however, most begin the weaning process between the time their baby is six to nine months old. Many babies make the decision for themselves, and begin to lose interest in nursing. Others may need a bit of encouragement.

Don't try to wean your baby from the breast while the little one is making other adjustments. If your baby resists weaning at first, and this is quite possible, postpone it for a week or two before trying again. Overcoaxing may only compound the problem.

How you handle weaning your breastfed baby is considerably more important than when you do it. Whether you realize it or not, weaning is going to be rough on both of you. For all this time, you have been the sole provider of your baby's life needs— the source of health and comfort. Now suddenly this relationship is being shaken; the strong bonds of dependence are weakened just a bit. While your baby can't dwell on these changes as you can, your child is very aware that they are taking place. Baby can sense that something is wrong or different and may not know how to react.

To avoid a great deal of heart-wrenching, start weaning gradually. Cut back one feeding at a time until your baby has stopped nursing entirely. But while you are reducing your milk, don't reduce the amount of affection you give. Your baby needs more love and attention now than ever—and so do you. Your whole family can ease the transitional period by lavishing more care on both members of the nursing couple.

You've done your best to provide a good start; now it's time for baby to inch out, bit by bit, and start to become an independent little person. Feel proud—your child is growing up.

Weaning the Natural Way

Natural weaning is slow and gradual. Sometimes your baby won't be interested in nursing; other times you may be busy and find that your infant has fallen asleep before you've had a chance to breastfeed. Slowly, one feeding and then another is missed until your baby is self-sufficient where eating is concerned. This process may take a few weeks or several months. You and your baby must set the pace that's right for you.

Making a Schedule. As we've said, begin weaning by eliminating one breastfeeding at a time. Try starting with the mid-afternoon feeding. Instead of offering your breast, give your baby some formula instead. Cow's milk and skim and low-fat products are all unsuitable; they're too high in protein and sodium, difficult to digest, and deficient in iron, copper, and vitamin C. Do not express breast milk for these feedings or your supply will continue to build up.

Whether you wean to a bottle or directly to a cup will depend on your baby's age and capabilities. For younger babies under six months old, attempt to wean to a bottle first. If your baby refuses the nipple, try a cup. Weighted, two-handled training cups with spouts are available to help your baby along. Infant eating utensils are described more fully in *The Evenflo Guide to Preparing to Bring Baby Home.* When

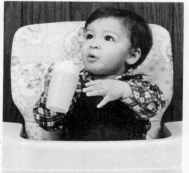

starting cup feeding, only fill about one-third of the cup until your baby becomes accustomed to the new sensation.

Several days or weeks later, drop out the midmorning feeding. The last feeding to go will probably be the early morning or late evening one when your baby needs the comfort and security of your breast the most. When you are down to just one feeding of breast milk daily, skip a day, then two days, and continue to increase the time between nursings. Soon your baby will lose interest in this uncertain proportion, maybe sucking for but a moment or two before finding some other means of satisfaction.

What if your baby becomes ill during the weaning period? To deny the comforts and relief of your breastfeeding on which baby has relied for so long is not a good idea. If this happens, it may be wiser to delay complete weaning until your baby is well.

All during the time, your milk supply will be on the decrease. Recall the breastfeeding law of supply and demand. Without the constant stimulus of your baby's sucking, your brain does not signal the production of the milk hormones. Because these changes occur over a period of time, though, you should experience little or no discomfort.

Sudden Weaning

Sudden weaning is stressful for both mother and child; it's much better to let nature take its course. But what if you must abruptly wean your breastfed infant because you must undergo surgery or have developed a serious illness? Your baby will have no choice but to become accustomed to the bottle, but may feel rejected. If you are unable to be with your baby during this period, your husband should make an effort to reassure the baby in your absence. No book says that a father can't "mother" a baby, too!

The rapid decrease in the demand for your breast milk will affect you as well. Expect to experience a few days discomfort from engorgement. Hand expressing a little milk or applying ice packs may bring some relief. If the problem continues, your doctor may prescribe hormones, often estrogen, to dry up your milk. If you are returning to the use of oral contraceptives, they may have a similar—though not as rapid—effect.

Weaning Affects You, Too

If you wean your baby naturally, your breasts will shrink back close to normal size by the end of the weaning period. Complete stoppage of your milk may take three or four months; you may find that you can still express a drop or two even if your baby has not been nursing for some time. Once the milk recedes totally, your breasts may feel a little less firm. This is not due to nursing, but to the weight you gained during pregnancy. If you have allotted enough time for proper breast care, this should not be a major worry.

Sudden weaning also brings an end to lactation, but not as smoothly. For the first few days, your breasts will continue to fill with milk as if you were nursing full time. This is the cause of the discomfort we've mentioned. It will take time for your breasts to empty, perhaps up to six months.

Emotional Aftermath. Your emotional reaction to weaning your baby may be more severe than any physical effects you may have to weather. Once milk production stops, your normal hormonal balance switches back to its pre-pregnancy state. Many mothers undergo a sort of "postlactation" depression similar to the blues felt after birth. You may harbor a sense of grief or be lonely or depressed as if something vital has been taken out of your life. You may think that your baby is rejecting you, that your constant care is no longer warranted.

Weaning undoubtedly creates a major change in the relationship you've had with your baby since birth, but it is, at the same time, a natural step you must follow to help your child grow up. Though a nursing relationship is irreplaceable, there are many other ways you can show love for your baby. Parenting involves understanding and adapting to your baby's changing needs. Weaning is but one small part in this drift toward self-sufficiency and independence. And although you may feel sad or wistful that the loving times you experienced while breastfeeding are past, you and your husband have many, many more joyous events ahead of you. After all, your baby's life has only begun.